Minimally Invasive Urological Procedures and Related Technological Developments—Series 2

Minimally Invasive Urological Procedures and Related Technological Developments—Series 2

Editor

Bhaskar K Somani

MDPI • Basel • Beijing • Wuhan • Barcelona • Belgrade • Manchester • Tokyo • Cluj • Tianjin

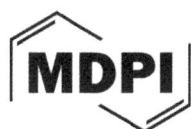

Editor
Bhaskar K Somani
Urological Surgery Department
University Hospital Southampton NHS
Foundation Trust
UK

Editorial Office
MDPI
St. Alban-Anlage 66
4052 Basel, Switzerland

This is a reprint of articles from the Special Issue published online in the open access journal *Journal of Clinical Medicine* (ISSN 2077-0383) (available at: https://www.mdpi.com/journal/jcm/special_issues/Minimally_Invasive_Urological_Procedures_2).

For citation purposes, cite each article independently as indicated on the article page online and as indicated below:

LastName, A.A.; LastName, B.B.; LastName, C.C. Article Title. *Journal Name* **Year**, *Volume Number*, Page Range.

ISBN 978-3-0365-7766-1 (Hbk)
ISBN 978-3-0365-7767-8 (PDF)

Cover image courtesy of Bhaskar K Somani.

© 2023 by the authors. Articles in this book are Open Access and distributed under the Creative Commons Attribution (CC BY) license, which allows users to download, copy and build upon published articles, as long as the author and publisher are properly credited, which ensures maximum dissemination and a wider impact of our publications.
The book as a whole is distributed by MDPI under the terms and conditions of the Creative Commons license CC BY-NC-ND.

Contents

About the Editor vii

Bhaskar Somani
Minimally Invasive Urological Procedures and Related Technological Developments—Series 2
Reprinted from: *J. Clin. Med.* **2023**, *12*, 2879, doi:10.3390/jcm12082879 1

Mriganka M. Sinha, Amelia Pietropaolo, Yesica Quiroz Madarriaga, Erika Llorens de Knecht, Anna Bujons Tur, Stephen Griffin and Bhaskar K. Somani
Comparison and Evaluation of Outcomes of Ureteroscopy and Stone Laser Fragmentation in Extremes of Age Groups (≤10 Years and ≥80 Years of Age): A Retrospective Comparative Analysis of over 15 Years from 2 Tertiary European Centres
Reprinted from: *J. Clin. Med.* **2023**, *12*, 1671, doi:10.3390/ jcm12041671 5

Zhongyi Li, Zhihuan Zheng, Xuesong Liu, Quan Zhu, Kaixuan Li, Li Huang, Zhao Wang and Zhengyan Tang
Venous Thromboembolism and Bleeding after Transurethral Resection of the Prostate (TURP) in Patients with Preoperative Antithrombotic Therapy: A Single-Center Study from a Tertiary Hospital in China
Reprinted from: *J. Clin. Med.* **2023**, *12*, 417, doi:10.3390/jcm12020417 13

Alba Sierra, Mariela Corrales, Bhaskar Somani and Olivier Traxer
Laser Efficiency and Laser Safety: Holmium YAG vs. Thulium Fiber Laser
Reprinted from: *J. Clin. Med.* **2023**, *12*, 149, doi:10.3390/jcm12010149 23

Alba Sierra, Mariela Corrales, Merkourios Kolvatzis, Steeve Doizi and Olivier Traxer
Real Time Intrarenal Pressure Control during Flexible Ureterorrenscopy Using a Vascular PressureWire: Pilot Study
Reprinted from: *J. Clin. Med.* **2023**, *12*, 147, doi:10.3390/jcm12010147 33

Vathsala Patil, Deepak Kumar Singhal, Nithesh Naik, B. M. Zeeshan Hameed, Milap J. Shah, Sufyan Ibrahim, Komal Smriti, et al.
Factors Affecting the Usage of Wearable Device Technology for Healthcare among Indian Adults: A Cross-Sectional Study
Reprinted from: *J. Clin. Med.* **2022**, *11*, 7019, doi:10.3390/jcm11237019 41

Yi-Yang Liu, Yen-Ta Chen, Hao-Lun Luo, Yuan-Chi Shen, Chien-Hsu Chen, Yao-Chi Chuang, Ko-Wei Huang, et al.
Totally X-ray-Free Ultrasound-Guided Mini-Percutaneous Nephrolithotomy in Galdakao-Modified Supine Valdivia Position: A Novel Combined Surgery
Reprinted from: *J. Clin. Med.* **2022**, *11*, 6644, doi:10.3390/jcm11226644 53

Kirolos G. F. T. Michael and Bhaskar K. Somani
Variation in Tap Water Mineral Content in the United Kingdom: Is It Relevant for Kidney Stone Disease?
Reprinted from: *J. Clin. Med.* **2022**, *11*, 5118, doi:10.3390/jcm11175118 63

Ziad H. Abd and Samir A. Muter
Comparison of the Safety and Efficacy of Laser Versus Pneumatic Intracorporeal Lithotripsy for Treatment of Bladder Stones in Children
Reprinted from: *J. Clin. Med.* **2022**, *11*, 513, doi:10.3390/jcm11030513 73

Vineet Gauhar, Daniele Castellani, Jeremy Yuen-Chun Teoh, Carlotta Nedbal, Giuseppe Chiacchio, Andrew T. Gabrielson, Flavio Lobo Heldwein, et al.
Catheter-Associated Urinary Infections and Consequences of Using Coated versus Non-Coated Urethral Catheters—Outcomes of a Systematic Review and Meta-Analysis of Randomized Trials
Reprinted from: *J. Clin. Med.* **2022**, *11*, 4463, doi:10.3390/jcm11154463 . . . . **81**

Vasileios Gkolezakis, Bhaskar Kumar Somani and Theodoros Tokas
Low- vs. High-Power Laser for Holmium Laser Enucleation of Prostate
Reprinted from: *J. Clin. Med.* **2023**, *12*, 2084, doi:10.3390/jcm12052084 . . . . **95**

Ee Jean Lim, Daniele Castellani, Wei Zheng So, Khi Yung Fong, Jing Qiu Li, Ho Yee Tiong, Nariman Gadzhiev, et al.
Radiomics in Urolithiasis: Systematic Review of Current Applications, Limitations, and Future Directions
Reprinted from: *J. Clin. Med.* **2022**, *11*, 5151, doi:10.3390/jcm11175151 . . . . **107**

About the Editor

Bhaskar K Somani

Bhaskar K Somani has been involved in clinically innovative patient-centred treatments. His research includes minimally invasive surgical techniques in the management of kidney stone disease, enlarged prostate (BPH), renal cancer and urinary tract infections. He is the Clinical Director of 'South Coast Lithotripter Services'. He is an active member of BAUS Endourology sub-section and is the Wessex Clinical Research Network and Simulation Lead for Urology. He is a board member of the European School of Urology (ESU), ESU Training and Research group and EAU section of the uro-technology (ESUT) endourology group. He is also the chosen representative for the UK in the Endourology society and is a member of the EAU urolithiasis guidelines panel. He coordinates the largest hands-on-training simulation course for urology in the world (EAU-EUREP). He has published over 550 scientific papers and has been invited as a speaker to perform live surgery for moderations in more than 30 countries worldwide. He has raised a grant income of GBP 3.2 million. He has published excellent clinical outcomes; his outcomes and research translate into benefits for patients. For his work, he has won the Endo Society 'Arthur Smith' award in 2020, BAUS 'Golden Telescope' in 2021 and Zenith Global Health Special Recognition award in 2021.

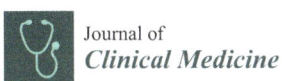

Editorial

Minimally Invasive Urological Procedures and Related Technological Developments—Series 2

Bhaskar Somani

Department of Urology, University Hospital Southampton NHS Foundation Trust, Southampton SO166YD, UK; bhaskarsomani@yahoo.com

The world of minimally invasive urology has experienced enormous growth in recent decades with technological innovations related to new techniques and equipment, better training, and the clinical adoption of translational research. There has been a substantial increase in studies related to the application of lasers both for the treatment of stones and enlarged prostates. This Special Issue in the *Journal of Clinical Medicine* (JCM) is dedicated to a collection of eleven high-quality scientific contributions.

The first paper looked at a systematic review and meta-analysis of randomised trials on the use of coated versus non-coated urethral catheters for the prevention of catheter-associated urinary tract infections (CAUTI) [1]. A meta-analysis of 12 studies and 36,783 patients showed no significant difference in patients with long-term catheterization, and this benefit of coated catheters should be balanced against the cost to healthcare. The second paper compares the mineral content of tap water in UK and whether this was relevant to kidney stone disease (KSD) [2]. Data from 66 UK cities showed a significant variation, and depending on where someone lived, drinking 2–3 L of tap water could contribute over one-third of the recommended daily calcium and magnesium, with possible implications for KSD incidence and recurrence.

Lasers have evolved with the advent of high-power holmium lasers, thulium fiber laser (TFL), and pulse modulation such as Moses technology [3–5]. There are four papers involving the use of lasers in endourology [6–10]. Laser efficiency and safety were compared between Holmium YAG and TFL lasers, with the latter showing higher efficiency [6]. Laser lithotripsy during ureteroscopy and stone fragmentation with comparative outcomes between ≤10 years and ≥80 years were examined by the second paper [7]. The results showed that while the former group had a higher incidence of repeated procedure, there was no difference in the overall stone-free rate (SFR) and complications between the groups. The third paper looks at low- vs. high-power lasers during the Holmium laser enucleation of the prostate (HoLEP) procedure [8]. Current evidence shows no difference in outcomes between the two and that low-power HoLEP is safe, feasible, and effective. The last paper looked at a comparison of the safety and efficacy of laser vs. pneumatic intracorporeal lithotripsy for the treatment of bladder stones in children [9]. In this prospective randomised study of 64 children, while the stone treatment was similar between groups, pneumatic lithotripsy was associated with a significantly greater risk of having at least 1 adverse effect.

Fluoroless endourology has been on the rise to minimise radiation doses. The total X-ray-free ultrasound-guided mini-PCNL in a Galdakao-modified supine Valdivia position was reported in the next paper from Taiwan on 150 patients [10]. The outcomes show that complete X-ray procedures are feasible, safe, and effective. Intrarenal pressure monitoring is also postulated to help minimise complications, but so far, there was a lack of pressure monitoring devices [11,12]. Measuring and minimising pressure would lower the risk of sepsis and other related complications [13]. Real-time intrarenal pressure control during flexible ureteorenoscopy was demonstrated in the next study using a vascular wire [14]. In this pilot study, a pressure wire was placed in the renal cavities to measure the intrapelvic

Citation: Somani, B. Minimally Invasive Urological Procedures and Related Technological Developments—Series 2. *J. Clin. Med.* **2023**, *12*, 2879. https://doi.org/10.3390/jcm12082879

Received: 5 April 2023
Accepted: 10 April 2023
Published: 14 April 2023

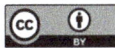

Copyright: © 2023 by the author. Licensee MDPI, Basel, Switzerland. This article is an open access article distributed under the terms and conditions of the Creative Commons Attribution (CC BY) license (https://creativecommons.org/licenses/by/4.0/).

pressure (IPP), with results showing the feasibility of this technique and the monitoring of IPP to identify and avoid high IPP, thereby avoiding complications.

In the world of smart apps [15], there is a rise in wearable device technology with an annual growth rate of nearly 26% projected for India. A cross-sectional web-based survey of 495 responders exhibited a significant correlation with the adoption and acceptance of wearable devices for healthcare management in the Indian context [16]. Minimally invasive surgical therapies (MISTs) for benign prostate enlargement (BPE) have experienced a revolution with new technologies that are now on the market [17–19]. However, the transurethral resection of prostate (TURP) is still practiced as the primary modality of treatments in many centres. In the context of cardiovascular morbidity, patients often have to remain with the choice of preoperative antithrombotic therapy. A single-centre study from China examined venous thromboembolism (VTE) and bleeding after TURP in patients with preoperative antithrombotic therapy [20]. In a cohort of 31 patients, the authors conclude that the short-term preoperative discontinuation of therapy may help patients obtain a relatively safe opportunity for TURP surgery. This must be balanced against the risks of VTE, perioperative bleeding, and serious cardiovascular and cerebrovascular complications.

Artificial intelligence (AI) is now used in various urological conditions, including urolithiasis, benign prostate hyperplasia (BPH), and uro-oncology [21]. Similarly, radiomics is increasingly applied to the diagnosis, management, and outcome prediction of various urological conditions [22]. In a systemic review of the role of radiomics in urolithiasis, seven studies were included [23], with radiomics used to identify calculi, differentiate phleboliths, and classify stone types and compositions pre-operatively. It has also been utilized to predict outcomes and complications after endourological procedures and, hence, has great future potential.

This Special Issue has several interesting papers that will help clinicians in decision making and treatment choices. While there is a spectrum of papers from tap water to catheters, lasers and its use in BPH and stone surgery, wearable devices, and the role of radiomics, perhaps more needs to be performed to address other aspects of a patient's journey, such as cost and the quality of life in the management of these patients [24,25]. I am thankful to the reviewers for their professional comments and to the *JCM* team for their ongoing support with this Special Issue. Lastly, I want to thank all authors for their valuable contributions.

Conflicts of Interest: The authors declare no conflict of interest.

References

1. Gauhar, V.; Castellani, D.; Teoh, J.Y.; Nedbal, C.; Chiacchio, G.; Gabrielson, A.T.; Heldwein, F.L.; Wroclawski, M.L.; de la Rosette, J.; Donalisio da Silva, R.; et al. Catheter-Associated Urinary Infections and Consequences of Using Coated versus Non-Coated Urethral Catheters—Outcomes of a Systematic Review and Meta-Analysis of Randomized Trials. *J. Clin. Med.* **2022**, *11*, 4463. [CrossRef]
2. Kirolos, G.F.T.M.; Somani, B.K. Variation in Tap Water Mineral Content in the United Kingdom: Is It Relevant for Kidney Stone Disease? *J. Clin. Med.* **2022**, *11*, 5118.
3. Pietropaolo, A.; Mani, M.; Hughes, T.; Somani, B.K. Role of low- *versus* high-power laser in the treatment of lower pole stones: Prospective non-randomized outcomes from a university teaching hospital. *Ther. Adv. Urol.* **2022**, *14*, 17562872221097345. [CrossRef]
4. Schembri, M.; Sahu, J.; Aboumarzouk, O.; Pietropaolo, A.; Somani, B.K. Thulium fiber laser: The new kid on the block. *Turk. J. Urol.* **2020**, *46* (Suppl. 1), S1–S10. [CrossRef]
5. Pietropaolo, A.; Jones, P.; Whitehurst, L.; Somani, B.K. Role of 'dusting and pop-dusting' using a high-powered (100 W) laser machine in the treatment of large stones ($\geq$15 mm): Prospective outcomes over 16 months. *Urolithiasis* **2019**, *47*, 391–394. [CrossRef]
6. Sierra, A.; Corrales, M.; Somani, B.; Traxer, O. Laser Efficiency and Laser Safety: Holmium YAG vs. Thulium Fiber Laser. *J. Clin. Med.* **2022**, *12*, 149. [CrossRef]
7. Sinha, M.M.; Pietropaolo, A.; Madarriaga, Y.Q.; de Knecht, E.L.; Tur, A.B.; Griffin, S.; Somani, B.K. Comparison and Evaluation of Outcomes of Ureteroscopy and Stone Laser Fragmentation in Extremes of Age Groups ($\leq$10 Years and $\geq$80 Years of Age): A Retrospective Comparative Analysis of over 15 Years from 2 Tertiary European Centres. *J. Clin. Med.* **2023**, *12*, 1671. [CrossRef]
8. Gkolezakis, V.; Somani, B.K.; Tokas, T. Low- vs. High-Power Laser for Holmium Laser Enucleation of Prostate. *J. Clin. Med.* **2023**, *12*, 2084. [CrossRef]

9. Abd, Z.H.; Muter, S.A. Comparison of the Safety and Efficacy of Laser Versus Pneumatic Intracorporeal Lithotripsy for Treatment of Bladder Stones in Children. *J. Clin. Med.* **2022**, *11*, 513. [CrossRef]
10. Liu, Y.Y.; Chen, Y.T.; Luo, H.L.; Shen, Y.C.; Chen, C.H.; Chuang, Y.C.; Huang, K.W.; Wang, H.J. Totally X-ray-Free Ultrasound-Guided Mini-Percutaneous Nephrolithotomy in Galdakao-Modified Supine Valdivia Position: A Novel Combined Surgery. *J. Clin. Med.* **2022**, *11*, 6644. [CrossRef]
11. Whitehurst, L.A.; Somani, B.K. Perirenal haematoma after Ureteroscopy: A Systematic review. *J. Endourol.* **2017**, *31*, 438–445. [CrossRef]
12. Whitehurst, L.; Jones, P.; Somani, B.K. Mortality from kidney stone disease (KSD) as reported in the literature over the last two decades: A systematic review. *WJU* **2019**, *37*, 759–776. [CrossRef]
13. Chugh, S.; Pietropaolo, A.; Montanari, E.; Sarica, K.; Somani, B.K. Predictors of Urinary Infections and Urosepsis After Ureteroscopy for Stone Disease: A Systematic Review from EAU Section of Urolithiasis (EULIS). *Curr. Urol. Rep.* **2020**, *21*, 16. [CrossRef]
14. Sierra, A.; Corrales, M.; Kolvatzis, M.; Doizi, S.; Traxer, O. Real Time Intrarenal Pressure Control during Flexible Ureterorrenscopy Using a Vascular PressureWire: Pilot Study. *J. Clin. Med.* **2022**, *12*, 147. [CrossRef]
15. Jamnadass, E.; Aboumarzouk, O.; Kallidonis, P.; Emiliani, E.; Tailly, T.; Hruby, S.; Sanguedolce, F.; Atis, G.; Ozsoy, M.; Greco, F.; et al. The Role of Social Media and Internet Search Engines in Information Provision and Dissemination to Patients with Kidney Stone Disease: A Systematic Review from European Association of Urologists Young Academic Urologists. *J. Endourol.* **2018**, *32*, 673–684. [CrossRef]
16. Patil, V.; Singhal, D.K.; Naik, N.; Hameed, B.M.Z.; Shah, M.J.; Ibrahim, S.; Smrit, K.; Chatterjee, G.; Kale, A.; Sharma, A.; et al. Factors Affecting the Usage of Wearable Device Technology for Healthcare among Indian Adults: A Cross-Sectional Study. *J. Clin. Med.* **2022**, *11*, 7019. [CrossRef]
17. Westwood, J.; Geraghty, R.; Jones, P.; Rai, B.P.; Somani, B.K. Rezum: A new transurethral water vapour therapy for benign prostatic hyperplasia. *Ther. Adv. Urol.* **2018**, *10*, 327–333. [CrossRef]
18. Jones, P.; Rajkumar, G.N.; Rai, B.P.; Aboumarzouk, O.M.; Cleaveland, P.; Srirangam, S.J.; Somani, B.K. Medium-term outcomes of Urolift (minimum 12 months follow-up): Evidence from a systematic review. *Urology* **2016**, *97*, 20–24. [CrossRef]
19. Maclean, D.; Harris, M.; Drake, T.; Maher, B.; Modi, S.; Dyer, J.; Somani, B.; Hacking, N.; Bryant, T. Factors predicting a good symptomatic outcome after prostate artery embolization (PAE). *Cardiovasc. Interv. Radiol.* **2018**, *41*, 1152–1159. [CrossRef]
20. Li, Z.; Zheng, Z.; Liu, X.; Zhu, Q.; Li, K.; Huang, L.; Wang, Z.; Tang, Z. Venous Thromboembolism and Bleeding after Transurethral Resection of the Prostate (TURP) in Patients with Preoperative Antithrombotic Therapy: A Single-Center Study from a Tertiary Hospital in China. *J. Clin. Med.* **2023**, *12*, 417. [CrossRef]
21. Shah, M.; Naik, N.; Somani, B.K.; Hameed, B.M.Z. Artificial intelligence (AI) in urology—Current use and future directions. An iTRUE study. *Turk. J. Urol.* **2020**, *46* (Suppl. 1), S27–S39. [CrossRef]
22. Chiacchio, G.; Castellani, D.; Nedbal, C.; De Stefano, V.; Brocca, C.; Tramanzoli, P.; Galosi, A.B.; Donalisio da Silva, R.; Teoh, J.Y.-C.; Tiong, H.Y.; et al. Radiomics vs radiologist in prostate cancer. Results from a systematic review. *World J. Urol.* **2023**, *41*, 709–724. [CrossRef]
23. Lim, E.J.; Castellani, D.; So, W.Z.; Fong, K.Y.; Li, J.Q.; Tiong, H.Y.; Gadzhiev, N.; Heng, C.T.; Teoh, J.Y.-C.; Naik, N.; et al. Radiomics in Urolithiasis: Systematic Review of Current Applications, Limitations, and Future Directions. *J. Clin. Med.* **2022**, *11*, 5151. [CrossRef]
24. Chapman, R.A.; Somani, B.K.; Robertson, A.; Healy, S.; Kata, S.G. Decreasing cost of flexible ureterorenoscopy: Single-use laser fiber cost analysis. *Urology* **2014**, *83*, 1003–1005. [CrossRef]
25. Mehmi, A.; Jones, P.; Somani, B.K. Current status and role of patient-reported outcome measures (PROMs) in Endourology. *Urology* **2021**, *148*, 26–31. [CrossRef]

Disclaimer/Publisher's Note: The statements, opinions and data contained in all publications are solely those of the individual author(s) and contributor(s) and not of MDPI and/or the editor(s). MDPI and/or the editor(s) disclaim responsibility for any injury to people or property resulting from any ideas, methods, instructions or products referred to in the content.

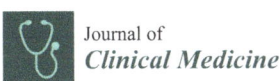

Article

Comparison and Evaluation of Outcomes of Ureteroscopy and Stone Laser Fragmentation in Extremes of Age Groups (≤10 Years and ≥80 Years of Age): A Retrospective Comparative Analysis of over 15 Years from 2 Tertiary European Centres

Mriganka M. Sinha [1], Amelia Pietropaolo [1], Yesica Quiroz Madarriaga [2], Erika Llorens de Knecht [3], Anna Bujons Tur [2], Stephen Griffin [3] and Bhaskar K. Somani [1,*]

[1] Urology Department, University Hospital Southampton NHS Trust, Southampton SO16 6YD, UK
[2] Pediatric Urology Unit, Urology Department, Fundació Puigvert, 08025 Barcelona, Spain
[3] Southampton Children Hospital NHS Trust, Southampton SO16 6YD, UK
* Correspondence: bhaskarsomani@yahoo.com

Abstract: Aim: To assess and compare the outcomes associated with ureteroscopy and laser fragmentation (URSL) for extremes of age group (≤10 and ≥80 years). Methods: Retrospective consecutive data were collected from two European centres for all paediatric patients ≤10 undergoing URSL over a 15-year period (group 1). It was compared to consecutive data for all patients ≥80 years (group 2). Data were collected for patient demographics, stone characteristics, operative details, and clinical outcomes. Results: A total of 168 patients had 201 URSL procedures during this time (74 and 94 patients in groups 1 and 2 respectively). The mean age and stone sizes were 6.1 years and 85 years, and 9.7 mm and 13 mm for groups 1 and 2 respectively. While the SFR was slightly higher in group 2 (92.5% versus 87.8%, $p = 0.301$), post-operative stent rate was also significantly higher in the geriatric population (75.9% versus 41.2%, $p = 0.0001$). There was also no significant difference in pre-operative stenting ($p = 0.886$), ureteric access sheath use (UAS) ($p = 0.220$) and post-operative complications. Group 1 had an intervention rate of 1.3/patient as compared to 1.1/patient in group 2. The overall complications were 7.2% and 15.3% in groups 1 and 2 respectively (0.069), with 1 Clavien IV complication related to post-operative sepsis and brief ICU admission in group 2. Conclusion: The paediatric population had a marginally higher incidence of repeat procedure, but the overall SFR and complications were similar, and post-operative stent insertion rates were much better compared to geriatric patients. URSL is a safe procedure in the extremes of age groups with no difference in the overall outcomes between the two groups.

Keywords: ureteroscopy; laser; kidney calculi; paediatric; urolithiasis; stent; elderly

1. Introduction

The global trend in lifetime prevalence of kidney stone disease (KSD) has increased from 10% to 14% in the last two decades [1–3]. The European Association of Urology (EAU) [4] in their 2021 guidelines recommend flexible ureteroscopy and lasertripsy (FURSL) as the first line of treatment in adults for uncomplicated ureteric and renal stones measuring less than 2 cm.

Surgical interventions such as FURSL can be associated with possible side effects and complications that are greatly dependent on patient age and comorbidities. Paediatric patients with renal tract calculi commonly have congenital anatomical abnormality and/or recurrent UTI and often benefit from smaller instruments. In recent years, the incidence of KSD in the paediatric population appears to be increasing [2]. Advances in ureteroscopic technology have allowed ureteroscopy to be adapted to the paediatric population [5]. Miniaturised ureteroscopes with sizes as small as 4.5 Fr have been created for paediatric cases to help improve the surgical outcome with minimal ureteral trauma [6]. These replace the historical 8.5/9.5 and 11 Fr scopes used in adults [7] The existing evidence for paediatric ureteroscopy for stone disease has demonstrated stone free rates (SFR) ranging between 58 and 100% [8,9] and low risk of complications; mainly Clavien–Dindo grade I–II [8].

Age progression towards geriatric population brings with it an entire cohort of physiological, anatomical and molecular changes. These translate into elderly patients presenting with multiple co-morbidities, possibly with pre-existing urinary symptoms requiring longer length of stay and more susceptible to general anaesthetic-associated complications [10]. Due to the increasing prevalence of KSD and need for intervention in both paediatric and geriatric age groups, we conducted this comparative retrospective analysis for these cohorts, and assessed the outcomes of FURSL, to evaluate its safety and efficacy in these two specific patient groups in the extremes of age groups ($\leq$10 years and $\geq$80 years of age).

2. Materials and Methods

Retrospective data for consecutive paediatric procedures for patients $\leq$10 years of age from two tertiary paediatric endourological European centres (University Hospital Southampton, United Kingdom and Fundació Puigvert hospital, Spain) operating independently of each other were collected and analysed. This study was registered locally as an audit in University Hospital Southampton (audit number 6901) and was approved by the ethics committee in Fundació Puigvert hospital wherein all parents were consented for participation in the study. This was compared with retrospectively collected data for consecutive geriatric patients ($\geq$80 years old) from the UK adult tertiary Endourological centre. The study was registered locally as an audit (audit number 6901) at University Hospital Southampton. The Fundació Puigvert hospital CEIM approved this study and family consent was obtained for all patients included in the study. The study period for the paediatric patients was from 2006–2021 (15 years) and adult patients from 2012–2021 (10 years).

A total of 201 FURSLs (168 patients) were performed in this time duration on 74 paediatric patients (group 1) and 94 geriatric patients (group 2). Data including age, gender, co-morbidities, American Society of Anaesthetics grading (ASA), symptom at time of presentation, laterality, stone size, site and biochemistry, date of surgery, duration of surgery, use of ureteric access sheath (UAS), pre and post-operative stent insertion, intra-operative and post-operative complications, stone free status, length of stay and follow-up were recorded. An intra-operative finding of being endoscopically stone free with post-operative imaging of fragments <2 mm was considered stone free.

The procedures were performed by experienced endourologists in both centres, and the data were collected independently by members of team not involved in the original procedure. Procedural details have been discussed and extensively detailed in the past (11–13). The diagnosis of stones was made by ultrasound scan (USS) and/or plain KUB XR, and non-contrast CT (NCCT) for groups 1 and 2 respectively. A follow-up USS was carried out for group 1 and a combination of USS (radiolucent stone) or KUB XR (radiopaque stone) or rarely NCCT (equivocal scan or persisting symptoms) for group 2 within 3 months of FURSL. A 4.5–6 F (Richard Wolf) semirigid scope and a 6 F (Storz) scope were used for groups 1 and 2 respectively. A Storz Flex X2 flexible ureteroscope [Karl Storz Endoscopy Ltd., Berkshire, UK] was used for all patients and while a 9.5/11.5 F ureteral access sheath (UAS) was used for group 1, a combination of 9.5/11.5 F or 12/14 F UAS was used for group 2. A Holmium:YAG laser [100 W, 60 W or 20 W Lumenis] was used for fragmentation using a 272-micron laser fibre (Lumenis, Inc., Santa Clara, CA, USA). Use of intra-operative UAS and post-operative stent was surgeon-dependent, and extracted stones were sent for crystallographic analysis.

Data were analysed and compared between the groups in terms of stone free rate, UAS use, stent use, complications and need for re-intervention. The data were initially collected in excel sheet (Microsoft, Redmond, WA, USA) and then anonymised and analysed in SPSS (IBM SPSS version 27). p-value was determined using chi-square test in SPSS for

3. Results

A total of 74 paediatric patients (group 1) and 94 geriatric patients (group 2) underwent 201 FURSL procedures during the study duration. The mean age and mean stone size for groups 1 and 2 was 6.1 years (range: 0.8–10 years) and 9.7 mm (range: 3–30 mm), and 85 years (range: 80–94 years) and 13 mm (range: 4–48 mm) respectively. The male: female ratio in group 1 was 1.4:1 vs. 2.4:1 in group 2 (Table 1).

Table 1. Patient demographics in both patient cohorts undergoing FURSL (PUJ—pelvi-ureteric junction, VUJ—vesico-ureteric junction, NOS—not otherwise specified, ICU—intensive care unit and CD—Clavien–Dindo complication grade).

Demographics	Paediatric Group (≤10 Years)	Geriatric Group (≥80 Years)
Number of patients	74	94
Number of procedures	97	104
Procedure: patient	1.3:1	1.1:1
Mean age +/−SD (Range)	6.1 ± 2.4 (Range: 0.8–10 years)	85 ± 3.9 (Range: 80–94 years)
Male: Female	1.4:1	2.4:1
Mean stone size +/−SD (Range) in mm	9.7 ± 4.4 (3–30)	13 ± 8.2 (4–48)
Stone location-Ureteric: Renal (Multiple stones)	1:1.2 (35)	1.2:1 (25)
Renal pelvis	23	7
Upper renal pole	13	7
Middle renal pole	18	15
Lower renal pole	35	19
Proximal ureter/PUJ	4	11
Mid ureter	3	15
Distal ureter/VUJ	25	28
NOS	11	15
Stone Biochemistry		
Calcium Oxalate	2	34
Struvite	4	2
Calcium Phosphate	3	0
Cystine	3	0
Uric acid	0	2
Mixed biochemistry	1	37
Unspecified	23	10

A UAS was used in 19.5% and 25.9% in groups 1 and 2 respectively. While the rate of pre- and post-operative stent rates were 42.2% and 41.2% in group 1, it was 43.2% and 75.9% in group 2. The SFR was found to be marginally better in group 2 with a SFR of 92.5% vs. 87.8% in group 1 ($p = 0.3$). There were three minor ureteric injury in group 1 which were all managed conservatively with a ureteric stent, with no recorded intra-operative complications in group 2. Marginal differences were noted in post-operative complications between group 1 (7.2%) and group 2 (15.3%) ($p = 0.069$). The complications for group 1 were all Clavien–Dindo I/II and ranged from UTI/sepsis ($n = 4$), haematuria ($n = 1$), urinary retention and catheterisation ($n = 2$). The complications for group 2 were UTI/sepsis ($n = 12$), haematuria ($n = 1$), urinary retention and catheterisation ($n = 1$), temporary acute kidney injury ($n = 1$) and sepsis needing ICU admission ($n = 1$). These findings are enlisted in Table 2. The operative time for group 1 was 83.9 ± 42.2 mins vs. 47.06 ± 25.7 mins in group 2, which reflects the way in which the operative time was calculated. While group 1 included anaesthetic time as well as procedural time, group 2 only included the procedural time. The most common stone biochemistry in group 1 was found to be struvite stones while in group 2 was calcium oxalate stones. Only 36 out of 74 patients in group 1 had stone analysis as opposed to 85 out of 94 in group 2, therefore no statistical analysis has been performed for the stone biochemistry.

Table 2. Intra-operative and post-operative outcomes of FURSL for both groups (CD—Clavien–Dindo classification of post-operative complications, UTI—urinary tract infection, ICU—intensive care unit, and AKI—acute kidney injury).

Details Compared	Paediatric Group (≤10 Years)	Geriatric Group (≥80 Years)	p Value
Duration of Surgery +/−SD	83.9 ± 42.2 mins	47.06 ± 25.7 mins	
Ureteric access sheath (UAS) use	19 (19.5%)	27 (25.9%)	0.220
Pre-operative stent	41/97 (42.2%)	45/104 (43.2%)	0.886
Post-operative stent	40/97 (41.2%)	79/104 (75.9%)	0.000
Stone free rate	87.8%	92.5%	0.301
Mean length of stay +/−SD (Range) in days	1.5 ± 1.7 (1–12)	0 ± 7.1 (0–61)	
Number of interventions/patient	1.3:1	1.1:1	
Complications			
Intra-operative			
Ureteric injury (stent inserted)	3	0	0.071
Post-operative			
Overall post-operative complications	7/97 (7.2%)	16/104 (15.3%)	0.069
Haematuria (CD)	1 (I)	1 (I)	0.960
UTI/sepsis	4 (II)	12 (II)	0.052
Sepsis requiring ICU admission	0	1 (IV)	0.333
Urine retention requiring catheterisation	2 (I)	1 (I)	0.520
Temporary AKI	0	1 (I)	0.333

The median length of stay (LOS) in group 1 was 1.5 days (range: 0–12 days) vs. 0 days (range: 0–61 days) in group 2. The number of interventions needed to achieve stone free status were 1.3 in group 1 and 1.1 in group 2. The patients were followed up in outpatient clinic with X-ray kidney-ureter-bladder (KUB), USSKUB or CTKUB.

4. Discussion

Our study demonstrates safety and efficacy of FURSL in patients at extremes of age groups. We found a SFR of 87.8% and 92.5% in group 1 and 2 respectively, which is comparable to the previously published data [9–14]. All ureteric injuries found in group 1 were minor and managed conservatively. While there was a difference in post-operative stent usage between the groups with higher usage in group 2, there was no significant difference between the SFR although group 1 had higher mean procedure/patient ratio to achieve this. Similarly, infection related complication was higher in group 2, which could potentially be a reflection of pre-operative lower urinary tract symptoms or incomplete bladder drainage, but this was not captured in our study.

In their study of 80 ureterorenoscopies published in 2014, Azili et al. [15] found a significant relationship between URS required in infancy and the need to convert to open surgery. However, with miniaturization of paediatric scopes, improved optics and technology, coupled with better training opportunities for operating surgeons, the need for invasive surgery can be further minimised. Somani et al. [16] have given useful insight into ways to improve surgical outcomes for paediatric URS including multi-disciplinary team approach for planning and management via a twin-surgeon technique and approach.

In their systematic review, Rob et al. [17] found an over-all complication rate for paediatric FURSL at 11.1%, with 31% Clavien–Dindo (CD) II and III complications. Conversely, our study showed an overall complication rate of 7.2% in group 1, with all Clavien I/II complications. We have not found an increase in complications in younger children undergoing

FURSL for kidney stones when compared against existing literature or against geriatric population [17], thereby reflecting safety of using FURSL for paediatric urolithiasis.

From the surgical point of view, FURSL is a minimally invasive procedure ensuring safety for this delicate patient cohort and the same efficacy provided as in adult patients can now be offered to paediatric patients [18]. Paediatric FURSL outcome has become superior to Extra-corporeal Shockwave Lithotripsy (ESWL) over the years [19]. In 2005, Tan et al. [20], mentioned the superiority of FURSL describing it as a first line option in stone treatment within the paediatric population. In a small patient group of 25 patients, they achieved a 95% SFR. These findings were confirmed by Thomas et al. [21]. More recently, Esposito et al. [22], compared the outcomes of FURSL between five paediatric high-volume centres finding a SFR of 97% and complication rates of 4%. Elsheemy et al. [23] in 2014 also analysed the outcome of 128 paediatric patients who underwent FURSL identifying that younger age and larger stones were predicting factors for post operative complications. However, a recent systematic review [17] underlined the importance of high volume experienced centres as a requirement for this type of specialist surgery and predictor of success.

At the other extreme of age, the geriatric population have different issues. These are often associated with general anaesthesia and possibly age related physiological and cognitive decline. The challenges due to age progression range from cardiovascular changes, presenting as higher blood pressures and reduced cardiac outputs, to decreased respiratory reserves due to suboptimal gas exchange along with reduced creatinine clearance and glomerular filtration causing renal dysfunction and poor drug elimination [24]. All the above, combined with increased susceptibility to post-operative confusion and delirium, refs. [24,25] require careful consideration and monitoring for GA administration in the geriatric population. Our study group had anaesthetic work up in preparation for surgery and careful consideration of anaesthetic and/or surgical needs in order to tailor them to the patients accordingly. Our median length of stay was 1.5 days in group 1 and 0 days in group 2 respectively, suggesting a quick recovery time in both these groups.

The definition of geriatric population in the literature is unclear [26] and ranged from over 65 years to over 75 years of age. Heyland et al. [27] in their prospective study of recovery after critical illness analysed 610 patients >80 years of age and found a significantly better outcome associated with younger age, lower frailty index and lower Charlson comorbidity score. They recommended assessment of frailty status and baseline physical function to improve outcomes in the elderly. In our study we found a 15.3% complication rate in the elderly with only one ICU admission for post-operative sepsis management. This is comparable to the existing evidence with 9% over-all complication rate found in patients >70 years of age by Prattley et al. [28] in their literature review of ureteroscopy for renal stone disease treatment. Emiliani et al. [29] compared the outcome of FURSL in both patients older and younger than 80 years old in a retrospective study. They found that despite the higher rate of comorbidity in the >80 patients' group, the SFR and complication rate were similar, but the operative time and hospital stay were higher. It is recognised that elderly patients can more likely be affected by multiple comorbidities that often require them to be on long-term antiplatelet or anticoagulation medications. A multicentric study involving 31 centres and 9982 patients found that the risk of post operative hospitalization is increased in those taking antiplatelet therapy [30].

Berardinelli et al. [31] also analysed patients of different age groups defining elderly patient above 65 years of age. They found that despite showing a high Charlson comorbidity index compared to their younger counterpart, SFR, operative time and re-intervention rate did not show differences between the two groups. Equally, surgical and medical complication rates were similar between the two cohorts. Similar to our study, Tolga-Gulpinar et al. [13] subdivided their patients undergoing FURSL into multiple age groups. They found that overall complication rates in children were not statistically higher than in adult patients. Perioperative complications were not related to the age groups. Cakici et al. [32] also described elderly patients as above 60 years old and compared FURSL outcome between them and younger patients without identifying significant findings.

Technological advances have now made ureteroscopy a frontline treatment for patients with stone disease in high risk patients including those at extremes of age [33–35]. A large multicentric global study from eight centres show that while ureteroscopy is acceptable as a first-line intervention in paediatric population, complications are higher in patients <5 years of age [36]. While group 1 included anaesthetic time as well as procedural time, group 2 only included the procedural time.

Strengths, Limitations and Areas of Future Research

While our study includes consecutive patients for both groups, data analysis was retrospective in nature. Record keeping for procedural duration differed in the two groups in our study. While group 1 included anaesthetic time as well as procedural time, group 2 only included the procedural time. We therefore recommend that future studies standardise how procedural time is calculated. While the study includes patients from 2 centres, future prospective studies with more high-volume centres could lead to a more accurate comparison of outcome in various age groups and with different comorbidities. The stone free definition should also be standardised with more work focussed on both cost and quality of life [37,38]. A recent study has also recommended a paediatric ureteroscopy (P-URS) reporting checklist and nomogram to aid studies in how outcomes are reported [39,40].

5. Conclusions

In this study we found FURSL to be safe and effective for stone disease management with comparable SFR in both paediatric and geriatric cohorts despite the slightly higher rate of re-intervention in the paediatric age group. There was no significant difference in the use of UAS although significantly fewer paediatric patients were deemed to require a post-operative ureteral stent. The outcomes of our study show extremely favourable results of FURSL in extremes of age groups, and hence should be considered as a first line treatment for these patients.

Author Contributions: Study design/concept: B.K.S.; data collection: M.M.S., A.P., Y.Q.M. and E.L.d.K.; data analysis: M.M.S.; manuscript draft: M.M.S.; critical appraisal of manuscript: A.P., Y.Q.M. and E.L.d.K., A.B.T., S.G. and B.K.S. All authors have read and agreed to the published version of the manuscript.

Funding: No funding was received for this paper.

Institutional Review Board Statement: The study was conducted according to the guidelines of the Declaration of Helsinki, and audit approval (audit number 6901) was taken.

Informed Consent Statement: Informed consent was obtained from all subjects/parents involved in the study.

Data Availability Statement: As data are identifiable, they will not be made available as per ethical approval.

Acknowledgments: We would like to thank all of the hospitals and surgeons for contributing data.

Conflicts of Interest: The authors declare no conflict of interest.

References

1. Pietropaolo, A.; Proietti, S.; Geraghty, R.; Skolarikos, A.; Papatsoris, A.; Liatsikos, E.; Somani, B.K. Trends of 'urolithiasis: Interventions, simulation, and laser technology' over the last 16 years (2000–2015) as published in the literature (PubMed): A systematic review from European section of Uro-technology (ESUT). *WJU* **2017**, *35*, 1651–1658. [CrossRef] [PubMed]
2. Rukin, N.J.; Siddiqui, Z.A.; Chedgy, E.C.; Somani, B.K. Trends in Upper Tract Stone Disease in England: Evidence from the Hospital Episodes Statistics Database. *Urol. Int.* **2017**, *98*, 391–396. [CrossRef] [PubMed]
3. Geraghty, R.M.; Jones, P.; Somani, B.K.; Hajiha, M.; Smith, J.; Amasyali, A.S.; Groegler, J.; Shah, M.; Alsyouf, M.; Krause, A.; et al. Worldwide Trends of Urinary Stone Disease Treatment Over the Last Two Decades: A Systematic Review. *J. Endourol.* **2017**, *31*, 547–556. [CrossRef] [PubMed]

4. Skolarikos, A.; Neisius, A.; Petřík, A.; Somani, B.; Thomas, K.; Gambaro, G. EAU Guidelines on Interventional Treatment for Urolithiasis. Available online: https://d56bochluxqnz.cloudfront.net/documents/full-guideline/EAU-Guidelines-on-Urolithiasis-2022.pdf (accessed on 1 March 2022).
5. Ost, M.C.; Fox, P.J., Jr. Pediatric Ureteroscopy. *J. Endourol.* **2018**, *32* (Suppl. S1), S117–S118. [CrossRef] [PubMed]
6. Utanğaç, M.M.; Sancaktutar, A.A.; Tepeler, A. Micro-ureteroscopy for the treatment of distal ureteral calculi in children. *J. Pediatr. Surg.* **2017**, *52*, 512–516. [CrossRef] [PubMed]
7. Al Busaidy, S.S.; Prem, A.R.; Medhat, M. Paediatric ureteroscopy for ureteric calculi: A 4-year experience. *BJU Int.* **1997**, *80*, 797–801. [CrossRef]
8. Ishii, H.; Griffin, S.; Somani, B.K. Ureteroscopy for stone disease in the paediatric population: A systematic review. *BJU Int.* **2015**, *115*, 867–873. [CrossRef]
9. Jones, P.; Rob, S.; Griffin, S.; Somani, B.K. Outcomes of ureteroscopy (URS) for stone disease in the paediatric population: Results of over 100 URS procedures from a UK tertiary centre. *World J. Urol.* **2020**, *38*, 213–218. [CrossRef]
10. Chen, D.X.; Yang, L.; Ding, L.; Li, S.Y.; Na Qi, Y.; Li, Q. Perioperative outcomes in geriatric patients undergoing hip fracture surgery with different anesthesia techniques: A systematic review and meta-analysis. *Medicine* **2019**, *98*, e18220. [CrossRef]
11. Mosquera, L.; Pietropaolo, A.; Brewin, A.; Madarriaga, Y.; de Knecht, E.; Jones, P.; Bujons, A.; Griffin, S.; Somani, B. Safety and Outcomes of using ureteric access sheath (UAS) for treatment of Pediatric renal stones: Outcomes from 2 tertiary endourology centers. *Urology* **2021**, *157*, 222–226. [CrossRef]
12. Mosquera, L.; Pietropaolo, A.; Madarriaga, Y.Q.; de Knecht, E.L.; Jones, P.; Tur, A.B.; Griffin, S.; Somani, B.K. Is Flexible Ureteroscopy and Laser Lithotripsy the New Gold Standard for Pediatric Lower Pole Stones? Outcomes from Two Large European Tertiary Pediatric Endourology Centers. *J. Endourol.* **2021**, *35*, 1479–1482. [CrossRef] [PubMed]
13. Pietropaolo, A.; Jones, P.; Whitehurst, L.; Somani, B.K. Role of 'dusting and pop-dusting' using a high-powered (100 W) laser machine in the treatment of large stones ($\geq$ 15 mm): Prospective outcomes over 16 months. *Urolithiasis* **2019**, *47*, 391–394. [CrossRef]
14. Featherstone, N.C.; Somani, B.K.; Griffin, S.J. Ureteroscopy and laser stone fragmentation (URSL) for large (>1 cm) paediatric stones: Outcomes from a university teaching hospital. *J. Pediatr. Urol.* **2017**, *13*, 202.e1–202.e7. [CrossRef] [PubMed]
15. Azili, M.N.; Ozcan, F.; Tiryaki, T. Retrograde intrarenal surgery for the treatment of renal stones in children: Factors influencing stone clearance and complications. *J. Pediatr. Surg.* **2014**, *49*, 1161–1165. [CrossRef] [PubMed]
16. Somani, B.K.; Griffin, S. Ureteroscopy for paediatric calculi: The twin-surgeon model. *J. Pediatr. Urol.* **2018**, *14*, 73–74. [CrossRef] [PubMed]
17. Rob, S.; Jones, P.; Pietropaolo, A.; Griffin, S.; Somani, B.K. Ureteroscopy for Stone Disease in Paediatric Population is Safe and Effective in Medium-Volume and High-Volume Centres: Evidence from a Systematic Review. *Curr. Urol. Rep.* **2017**, *18*, 92. [CrossRef] [PubMed]
18. Reddy, P.P. Pediatric ureteroscopy. *Urol. Clin. North Am.* **2004**, *31*, 145–156. [CrossRef]
19. Minevich, E. Management of ureteric stone in pediatric patients. *Indian J. Urol.* **2010**, *26*, 564–567. [CrossRef]
20. Tan, A.H.H.; Al-Omar, M.; Denstedt, J.; Razvi, H. Ureteroscopy for pediatric urolithiasis: An evolving first-line therapy. *Urology* **2005**, *65*, 153–156. [CrossRef]
21. Thomas, J.C.; Demarco, R.T.; Donohoe, J.M.; Adams, M.C.; Brock, J.W.; Pope, J.C. Pediatric ureteroscopic stone management. *J. Urol.* **2005**, *174*, 1072–1074. [CrossRef]
22. Esposito, C.; Masieri, L.; Bagnara, V.; Tokar, B.; Golebiewski, A.; Escolino, M. Ureteroscopic lithotripsy for ureteral stones in children using holmium: Yag laser energy: Results of a multicentric survey. *J. Pediatr. Urol.* **2019**, *15*, 391.e1–391.e7. [CrossRef] [PubMed]
23. Elsheemy, M.S.; Maher, A.; Mursi, K.; Shouman, A.M.; Shoukry, A.I.; Morsi, H.A.; Meshref, A. Holmium:YAG laser ureteroscopic lithotripsy for ureteric calculi in children: Predictive factors for complications and success. *World J. Urol.* **2014**, *32*, 985–990. [CrossRef] [PubMed]
24. Alvis, B.D.; Hughes, C.G. Physiology Considerations in Geriatric Patients. *Anesthesiol. Clin.* **2015**, *33*, 447–456. [CrossRef] [PubMed]
25. Peters, R. Ageing and the brain. *Postgrad Med. J.* **2006**, *82*, 84–88. [CrossRef]
26. Singh, S.; Bajorek, B. Defining "elderly" in clinical practice guidelines for pharmacotherapy. *Pharm. Pr. (Internet)* **2014**, *12*, 489. [CrossRef]
27. Heyland, D.K.; Garland, A.; Bagshaw, S.M.; Cook, D.; Rockwood, K.; Stelfox, H.T.; Dodek, P.; Fowler, R.A.; Turgeon, A.F.; Burns, K.; et al. Recovery after critical illness in patients aged 80 years or older: A multi-center prospective observational cohort study. *Intensiv. Care Med.* **2015**, *41*, 1911–1920. [CrossRef]
28. Prattley, S.; Voss, J.; Cheung, S.; Geraghty, R.; Jones, P.; Somani, B.K. Ureteroscopy and stone treatment in the elderly ($\geq$70 years): Prospective outcomes over 5- years with a review of literature. *Int. Braz J. Urol* **2018**, *44*, 750–757. [CrossRef]
29. Emiliani, E.; Piccirilli, A.; Cepeda-Delgado, M.; Kanashiro, A.K.; Mantilla, D.; Amaya, C.A.; Sanchez-Martin, F.M.; Millan-Rodriguez, F.; Territo, A.; Amón-Sesmero, J.H.; et al. Flexible ureteroscopy in extreme elderly patients (80 years of age and older) is feasible and safe. *World J. Urol.* **2021**, *39*, 2703–2708. [CrossRef]

30. Hiller, S.C.; Qi, J.; Leavitt, D.; Frontera, J.R.; Jafri, S.M.; Hollingsworth, J.M.; Dauw, C.A.; Ghani, K.R. Ureteroscopy in Patients Taking Anticoagulant or Antiplatelet Therapy: Practice Patterns and Outcomes in a Surgical Collaborative. *J. Urol.* **2021**, *205*, 833–840. [CrossRef]
31. Berardinelli, F.; De Francesco, P.; Marchioni, M.; Cera, N.; Proietti, S.; Hennessey, D.; Dalpiaz, O.; Cracco, C.; Scoffone, C.; Giusti, G.; et al. RIRS in the elderly: Is it feasible and safe? *Int. J. Surg.* **2017**, *42*, 147–151. [CrossRef]
32. Cakici, M.C.; Sari, S.; Selmi, V.; Sandikci, F.; Karakoyunlu, N.; Ozok, U. Is the Efficacy and Safety of Retrograde Flexible Ureteroscopy in the Elderly Population Different from Non-elderly Adults? *Cureus* **2019**, *11*, e4852. [CrossRef] [PubMed]
33. Wright, A.E.; Rukin, N.J.; Somani, B.K. Ureteroscopy and stones: Current status and future expectations. *World J. Nephrol.* **2014**, *3*, 243–248. [CrossRef]
34. Somani, B.K.; Dellis, A.; Liatsikos, E.; Skolarikos, A. Review on diagnosis and management of urolithiasis in pregnancy: An ESUT practical guide for urologists. *World J. Urol.* **2017**, *35*, 1637–1649. [CrossRef] [PubMed]
35. Karim, S.S.; Hanna, L.; Geraghty, R.; Somani, B.K. Role of pelvicalyceal anatomy in the outcomes of retrograde intrarenal surgery (RIRS) for lower pole stones: Outcomes with a systematic review of literature. *Urolithiasis* **2020**, *48*, 263–270. [CrossRef] [PubMed]
36. Lim, E.J.; Traxer, O.; Madarriaga, Y.Q.; Castellani, D.; Fong, K.Y.; Chan, V.W.-S.; Tur, A.B.; Pietropaolo, A.; Ragoori, D.; Shrestha, A.; et al. Outcomes and lessons learnt from practice of retrograde intrarenal surgery (RIRS) in a paediatric setting of various age groups: A global study across 8 centres. *World J. Urol.* **2022**, *40*, 1223–1229. [CrossRef]
37. Somani, B.K.; Desai, M.; Traxer, O.; Lahme, S. Stone-free rate (SFR): A new proposal for defining levels of SFR. *Urolithiasis* **2014**, *42*, 95. [CrossRef]
38. Geraghty, R.M.; Jones, P.; Herrmann, T.R.W.; Aboumarzouk, O.; Somani, B.K. Ureteroscopy is more cost effective than shock wave lithotripsy for stone treatment: Systematic review and meta-analysis. *World J. Urol.* **2018**, *36*, 1783–1793. [CrossRef]
39. Brown, G.; Juliebø-Jones, P.; Keller, E.X.; De Coninck, V.; Beisland, C.; Somani, B.K. Current status of nomograms and scoring systems in paediatric endourology: A systematic review of literature. *J. Pediatr. Urol.* **2022**, *18*, 572–584. [CrossRef]
40. Juliebø-Jones, P.; Ulvik, Ø.; Beisland, C.; Somani, B.K. Paediatric Ureteroscopy (P-URS) reporting checklist: A new tool to aid studies report the essential items on paediatric ureteroscopy for stone disease. *Urolithaisis* **2023**, *51*, 35. [CrossRef]

Disclaimer/Publisher's Note: The statements, opinions and data contained in all publications are solely those of the individual author(s) and contributor(s) and not of MDPI and/or the editor(s). MDPI and/or the editor(s) disclaim responsibility for any injury to people or property resulting from any ideas, methods, instructions or products referred to in the content.

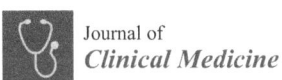

Article

Venous Thromboembolism and Bleeding after Transurethral Resection of the Prostate (TURP) in Patients with Preoperative Antithrombotic Therapy: A Single-Center Study from a Tertiary Hospital in China

Zhongyi Li [1], Zhihuan Zheng [1], Xuesong Liu [1], Quan Zhu [1], Kaixuan Li [1], Li Huang [2], Zhao Wang [1,*,†] and Zhengyan Tang [1,*,†]

[1] Department of Urology, Xiangya Hospital, Central South University, Changsha 410008, China
[2] Department of Critical Care Medicine, Xiangya Hospital, Central South University, Changsha 410008, China
* Correspondence: xywangz07@163.com (Z.W.); xytzyan@163.com (Z.T.)
† These authors contributed equally to this work.

Abstract: Background: Venous thromboembolism (VTE) and postoperative hemorrhage are unavoidable complications of transurethral resection of the prostate (TURP). At present, more and more patients with benign prostate hyperplasia (BPH) need long-term antithrombotic therapy before operation due to cardiovascular diseases or cerebrovascular diseases. The purpose of this study was to investigate the effect of preoperative antithrombotic therapy history on lower extremity VTE and bleeding after TURP. Methods: Patients who underwent TURP in the Department of Urology, Xiangya Hospital, Central South University, from January 2017 to December 2021 and took antithrombotic drugs before operation were retrospectively analyzed. The baseline data of patients were collected, including age, prostate volume, preoperative International Prostate Symptom Score (IPSS), complications, surgical history within one month, indications of preoperative antithrombotic drugs, drug types, medication duration, etc. Main outcome measures included venous thromboembolism after TURP, intraoperative and postoperative bleeding, and perioperative blood transfusion. Secondary outcome measures included operation duration and postoperative hospitalization days, the duration of stopping antithrombotic drugs before operation, the recovery time of antithrombotic drugs after operation, the condition of lower limbs within 3 months after operation, major adverse cardiac events (MACEs), and cerebrovascular complications and death. Results: A total of 31 patients after TURP with a long preoperative history of antithrombotic drugs were included in this study. Six patients (19.4%) developed superficial venous thrombosis (SVT) postoperatively. Four of these patients progressed to deep vein thrombosis (DVT) without pulmonary thromboembolism (PE). Only one patient underwent extra bladder irrigation due to blockage of their urinary catheter by a blood clot postoperatively. The symptoms of hematuria mostly disappeared within one month postoperatively and lasted for up to three months postoperatively. No blood transfusion, surgical intervention to stop bleeding, lower limb discomfort such as swelling, MACEs, cerebrovascular complications, or death occurred in all patients within three months after surgery. Conclusion: Short-term preoperative discontinuation may help patients with antithrombotic therapy to obtain a relatively safe opportunity for TURP surgery after professional evaluation of perioperative conditions. The risks of perioperative bleeding, VTE, and serious cardiovascular and cerebrovascular complications are relatively controllable. It is essential for urologists to pay more attention to the perioperative management of these patients. However, further high-quality research results are needed for more powerful verification.

Keywords: antithrombotic therapy; transurethral resection of the prostate; postoperative hemorrhage; venous thromboembolism

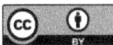

1. Introduction

Benign prostate hyperplasia (BPH) is a common urinary system disease in elderly men which greatly affects the quality of life for these patients. The clinical manifestations are mainly lower urinary tract symptoms (LUTS) such as frequent micturition, urgency, increased nocturia, weak micturition, incomplete urination, etc. Transurethral resection of the prostate (TURP) is the main surgical method for BPH patients, and its risks include postoperative bleeding and venous thromboembolism (VTE) [1–4]. VTE refers to deep vein thrombosis (DVT) and pulmonary thromboembolism (PE) [5]. However, superficial venous thrombosis (SVT) is more common in clinical practice [6].

The incidence of BPH increases with age. Many elderly patients need long-term antithrombotic therapy before surgery due to cardiovascular or cerebrovascular diseases [7]. Antithrombotic therapy includes anticoagulation and antiplatelet therapy. If antithrombotic therapy is discontinued during the perioperative period, the risk of cardiovascular and cerebrovascular events will increase [8], while continuing therapy will increase the risk of bleeding after TURP [9]. A previous study showed that the history of antithrombotic drug treatment within one month was an independent risk factor for VTE after urological non-malignant tumor surgery, and the risk of VTE after surgery was markedly increased 10-fold compared to that of patients without antithrombotic drug use [10]. The timing of preoperative discontinuation of antithrombotic drugs is critical. However, the existing studies [11,12] mostly focus on the influence of stopping time on postoperative hemorrhage risk and fail to comprehensively assess the risk of hemorrhage and VTE. In addition, most studies [13–15] only analyzed the effect of aspirin on TURP surgery, which is difficult to fully adapt to the actual complex clinical situation. Therefore, the purpose of this study is to explain the occurrence of VTE and bleeding after TURP in patients who stopped using antithrombotic drugs before operation, which may provide a reference for clinical practice.

2. Materials and Methods

2.1. Study Population

This study is a retrospective study and has been approved by the Ethics Committee of Xiangya Hospital of Central South University (No. 202011183). The inclusion criteria were as follows: (1) patients who underwent TURP surgery in the Department of Urology, Xiangya Hospital, Central South University, from January 2017 to December 2021; (2) duration for maintenance antithrombotic drugs before operation of more than one month. The following were exclusion criteria: (1) patients complicated with active malignant diseases; (2) a history of prostate surgery or urinary tract reconstruction surgery; (3) postoperative pathological examination showing prostate cancer; (4) VTE detected preoperatively; (5) bridging therapy such as low-molecular-weight heparin before operation.

According to the epidemiology and clinical symptoms of BPH patients, referring to the guidelines and experts' consensus on the prevention and treatment of BPH and VTE, the clinical data we collected mainly included age, prostate volume, preoperative International Prostate Symptom Score (IPSS), complications (hypertension, coronary heart disease, diabetes, stroke, varicose veins of lower limbs, etc.), surgical history within one month, and preoperative use of antithrombotic drugs.

2.2. Outcome Measures

The main outcomes are venous thromboembolism after TURP, intraoperative and postoperative bleeding, and perioperative blood transfusion. The amount of bleeding and the duration of the operation are all referred to in the surgical anesthesia record sheet. Postoperative bleeding can be divided into whether there is slight gross hematuria (reddish) or obvious gross hematuria (crimson) within 3 months after operation and whether extra bladder irrigation or re-operation is needed. Secondary outcomes include operation duration and postoperative hospitalization days, the duration of stopping antithrombotic drugs before operation, the recovery time of antithrombotic drugs after operation, the condition of the lower limbs, major adverse cardiac events (MACEs), cerebrovascular complications, and death within 3 months after operation. MACEs mainly mean acute myocardial infarction, cardiac arrest, severe arrhythmia, cardiac death, etc. Cerebrovascular complications mainly refer to stroke and transient ischemic attack.

2.3. Perioperative Management

In order to control the risk of perioperative bleeding, the patients who maintained antithrombotic therapy stopped taking antithrombotic drugs before TURP after evaluation and guidance by relevant specialists, and none of them used bridging therapy. After the risk of postoperative bleeding decreased, the original antithrombotic protocol was reactivated.

All patients were treated with mechanical thromboprophylaxis to prevent venous thromboembolism during the perioperative period. On the surgery day, patients were guided by specialized nurses to wear appropriate graduated compression stockings (GCS). The frequency of removing the graduated compression stockings was limited to three times a day, and the duration of removing time was limited to half an hour. Intermittent pneumatic compression (IPC) was applied after the postoperative patient returned to the ward [16].

Before and after the operation, the patients were examined by ultrasound in both lower limbs, which was performed by experienced sonographers. If a patient has postoperative symptoms such as dyspnea, syncope, hemoptysis, chest pain, shock, or decreased oxygen saturation, further examination such as pulmonary CTA and/or echocardiography is required to determine the occurrence of PE.

Once the patient was diagnosed with VTE or SVT, mechanical prevention of thrombosis (GCS and IPC) was immediately stopped according to the consultation opinion from the VTE group, and the risk of bleeding was assessed before anticoagulant therapy or even thrombolytic therapy immediately under the guidance of the VTE professional team.

2.4. Follow-Up

Follow-up was carried out at 7 days, 1 month, and 3 months after operation, mainly through outpatient service and telephone calls. The follow-up included drugs and the duration of prescription, hematuria or bleeding 3 months after surgery, lower extremity conditions, MACEs, cerebrovascular complications, and death.

2.5. Statistical Analysis

Data were analyzed using IBM SPSS 26.0 software. Quantitative data conforming to the normal distribution are expressed as mean ± standard deviation ($\bar{x} \pm s$), while those not conforming to the normal distribution are expressed as median (interquartile range). Qualitative data are expressed as cases (percentage) (n(%)).

3. Result

3.1. Patients' Baseline Data

A total of 31 patients who underwent TURP with a long history of taking antithrombotic drugs before operation (Table 1) were included in this study. The mean age of the 31 patients was 70.3 ± 6.5 years, the mean preoperative IPSS score was 20.2 ± 3.0, and the median prostate volume was 56.2 (44.9–85.6) mL. One patient (3.2%) underwent prostate biopsy within one month before TURP.

Among the 31 patients, 6 (19.4%) had coronary stent implantation, 2 (6.5%) had aortic valve replacement, 3 (9.7%) had mitral valve replacement, 2 (6.5%) had a history of myocardial infarction, 10 (32.3%) had a history of cerebral infarction, 6 (19.4%) had a history of coronary heart disease, and 2 (6.5%) had a history of atrial fibrillation. Two patients (6.5%) took long-term oral warfarin and twenty-nine patients (93.5%) took long-term oral antiplatelet drugs, including 19 patients (61.3%) taking aspirin, 6 patients (19.4%) taking clopidogrel, and 4 patients (12.9%) taking aspirin combined with clopidogrel. Three patients (9.7%) took medicine for less than one year, fifteen patients (48.4%) for 1–5 years, eleven patients (35.5%) for 5–10 years, and two patients (6.5%) for more than 10 years.

Table 1. Baseline information of patients and types, indications, and administration duration of antithrombotic drugs (n = 31).

	n (%)		n (%)
Age		Indications	
≥65 y	6 (19.4)	Coronary stent implantation	6 (19.4)
<65 y	25 (80.6)	Aortic valve replacement	2 (6.5)
Prostate volume		Mitral valve replacement	3 (9.7)
≤50 mL	13 (41.9)	Remote myocardial infarction	2 (6.5)
50–100 mL	16 (51.6)	Remote cerebral infarction	10 (32.3)
≥100 mL	2 (6.5)	Coronary heart disease	6 (19.4)
IPSS score		Atrial fibrillation	2 (6.5)
0–7	0 (0.0)	Drug information	
8–19	11 (35.5)	Aspirin	19 (61.3)
20–35	20 (64.5)	Clopidogrel	6 (19.4)
Operation history within 1 month	1 (3.2)	Aspirin and clopidogrel	4 (12.9)
Comorbidities		Warfarin	2 (6.5)
Hypertension	27 (87.1)	Medication duration	
Diabetes	5 (16.1)	≤1 year	3 (6.5)
Coronary heart disease	15 (48.4)	≤5 year	15 (48.4)
Apoplexy	16 (51.6)	≤10 year	11 (35.5)
Varicosity of lower limbs	1 (3.2)	>10 year	2 (6.5)

3.2. Incidence of VTE after TURP

SVT after surgery occurred in 6 (19.4%) of 31 TURP patients with a history of taking antithrombotic drugs preoperatively. Among them, four patients developed DVT without PE. In the remaining 25 patients, there was no SVT/DVT/PE (Table 2).

Table 2. Incidence of VTE after TURP (n = 31).

	n (%)
SVT	6 (19.4)
SVT only	*2 (6.5)*
SVT combined with DVT	*4 (12.9)*
SVT combined with PE	*0 (0.0)*
VTE (without SVT)	0 (0.0)
No VTE	25 (80.6)

3.3. Perioperative Situation of TURP

Among the 31 patients, antithrombotic drug discontinuation occurred in three cases (9.7%) within one week before surgery. In 24 cases (77.4%), the withdrawal time span was between one and two weeks, and in the other four cases (12.9%), it was more than two weeks. After preoperative drug discontinuation in 31 patients, no bridging therapy was performed and no new adverse events such as myocardial infarction and cerebral infarction occurred. The median operation duration was 75 (50–100) min, and the median intraoperative bleeding volume was 30 (10–100) mL. All patients were discharged 2–4 days after surgery, and nobody needed a blood transfusion during hospitalization (Table 3).

All patients were followed up at 7 days, 1 month, and 3 months after surgery. During the follow-up period, there was no lower extremity discomfort such as swelling, no MACEs, no cerebrovascular complications, and no death among all patients (Table 3). Two patients (6.5%) resumed antithrombotic therapy within 1 week after surgery. In 27 patients, the time for returning to antithrombotic drugs was between 1 week and 1 month after surgery. For the other two patients (6.5%), the resumption of postoperative antithrombotic regimens was delayed until 1 month later. Within 7 days after operation, reddish light hematuria was reported in 28 patients (90.3%). Crimson gross hematuria was reported in two patients, one of who was readmitted due to clot blockage of the catheter, and extra continuous bladder irrigation was performed to keep the catheter unobstructed. Within one month, 13 patients (41.9%) occasionally had reddish light hematuria. Only one patient with hematuria finally resolved after more than three months. None of the patients needed reoperation due to bleeding (Table 4).

Table 3. Perioperative conditions and clinical outcomes of TURP.

	n (%)
Preoperative withdrawal duration	
<1 week	3 (9.7)
1–2 week	24 (77.4)
>2 week	4 (12.9)
Pre-operation and post-withdrawal conditions	
New myocardial infarction	0 (0.0)
New cerebral infarction	0 (0.0)
Other new adverse events	0 (0.0)
Operation duration	
≤60 min	11 (35.5)
60–120 min	8 (25.8)
≥120 min	2 (6.5)
Intraoperative bleeding volume	
≤100 mL	28 (90.3)
100–400 mL	2 (6.5)
≥400 mL	1 (3.2)
Postoperative hospitalization days	
≤3 d	25 (80.6)
3–7 d	6 (19.4)
≥7 d	0 (0.0)
Time of postoperative antithrombotic recovery after operation	
<1 week	2 (6.5)
1 week–1 month after operation	27 (87.0)
>1 month after operation	2 (6.5)
Transfuse blood	0 (0.0)
Lower extremity discomfort	0 (0.0)
Postoperative MACEs	0 (0.0)
Cerebrovascular complications	0 (0.0)
Death	0 (0.0)

Table 4. Hemorrhage after TURP (n (%)).

Bleeding Conditions	Time	7 Days after Operation	7 Days–1 Month after Operation	1–3 Months after Operation
Reddish gross hematuria		28 (90.3)	13 (41.9)	1 (3.2)
Crimson gross hematuria		2 (6.5)	0 (0.0)	0 (0.0)
Bladder irrigation required		1 (3.2)	0 (0.0)	0 (0.0)
Reoperation required		0 (0.0)	0 (0.0)	0 (0.0)

4. Discussion

BPH is a common urination disorder in middle-aged and elderly men, and it is one of the most common diseases in the clinical practice of urology around the world. Approximately 50% of men over 60 years old are troubled by BPH, and about 30% eventually need surgery [17,18]. Many elderly patients with cardiovascular and cerebrovascular diseases need long-term oral antithrombotic drugs [7]. Studies have shown that roughly 4% of patients who need TURP take anticoagulants orally for a long time [19], and a larger proportion of patients take antiplatelet drugs [20].

Hemorrhage is an unavoidable complication after TURP [21–23]. If antithrombotics are used continuously during the perioperative period, the risk of surgical hemorrhage will be enlarged considerably. However, discontinuation of antithrombotics increases the incidence of adverse cardiovascular and cerebrovascular events [24]. The European Association of Urology (EAU) recommends that the timing of preoperative discontinuation of antithrombotic drugs in non-extremely high-risk patients should be adjusted according to the type of antithrombotic drug, ranging from 12 h before surgery (e.g., for unfractionated heparin) to 5–7 days (e.g., for clopidogrel) [25]. Dimitropoulos K et al. [12] suggested that oral antithrombotic therapy should be discontinued 7–10 days before TURP in patients with low risk of cardiovascular events. There is relatively much literature in this field regarding the effect of preoperative discontinuation of antithrombotic drugs on postoperative bleeding after TURP [14,26–28]. However, these studies have mainly focused on a single drug (aspirin) and a single complication (postoperative bleeding). Our study shows that patients taking aspirin antithrombotic therapy alone account for about 60% of all antithrombotic patients, which means that 40% of patients may still be taking other antithrombotic therapies, who lack evidence-based guidance for stopping antithrombotic drugs before TURP. After detailed questioning during hospitalization and follow-up within three months after discharge, it became apparent that most of the 31 patients included in this study had been instructed to discontinue antithrombotic drugs within 7 to 14 days before surgery. Only one patient underwent bladder irrigation due to a clogged urinary catheter with blood clot postoperatively. The symptoms of hematuria lasted for 3 months at most postoperatively. No patient underwent reoperation because of hemorrhage within 3 months postoperatively. Therefore, the risk of postoperative bleeding may be acceptable if antithrombotic drugs are temporarily stopped before operation, but it is obvious that large-scale and high-level evidence is still needed to clarify this.

VTE is also a common and potentially fatal complication after operation. As the third leading cause of cardiovascular death, it has received more and more attention from clinicians in recent years [29], and it is also one of the common perioperative complications of urological surgery. However, SVT is more common in clinical practice and has always been regarded as a benign self-limiting disease. One study showed that 18.1% of SVT patients were combined with DVT and 6.9% were combined with PE [30]. Obviously, the risk of SVT cannot be ignored [31,32]. Therefore, patients who underwent TURP surgery with postoperative SVT were included in this study. A previous study pointed out that taking antithrombotic drugs for a long time will affect the balance of the anticoagulation/coagulation system of the body. The discontinuation of antithrombotic drugs before TURP may make the body become hypercoagulable in a short time, thus increasing the probability of VTE postoperatively [10]. In our study, among the 31 patients who took antithrombotic drugs for a long time, six patients (18.9%) suffered from SVT or DVT after operation, which is much higher than the incidence of VTE after TURP in the normal elderly population (0.5–1.4%) [30,33]. However, it is similar to a previous research result [34]. Taking antithrombotic drugs may be a high risk factor for VTE after TURP, and there may be two reasons. First, discontinuation of antithrombotic drugs disrupts the long-term balance of the coagulation/anticoagulation system. Second, patients with BPH are mostly old men, and it is undeniable that aging is a risk factor for VTE.

In our study, although there were no serious complications such as pulmonary embolism, myocardial infarction, and cerebral infarction under active surveillance, the incidence of postoperative VTE in patients who stopped antithrombotic drugs before operation was significantly higher than that in the normal elderly population. Therefore, in clinical practice, it is still necessary to be highly alert to the risk of postoperative VTE in patients with previous antithrombotic therapy. Urologists need to raise awareness, actively monitor, and intervene in time.

Previous studies have focused on the effect of aspirin on bleeding after TURP, but as far as we know, there is a lack of research studying the effects of preoperative antithrombotic drug discontinuation on VTE after TURP. Our research takes both of them into account and expands the antithrombotic drugs from aspirin to various commonly used antithrombotic programs in clinics as well as exploring the discontinuation program of antithrombotic drugs with acceptable risk, which is more in line with the actual clinical situation. However, this study is a retrospective observational study, and it also has certain limitations. It cannot reveal the statistical difference in the incidence of VTE between patients treated with antithrombotic therapy and healthy elderly people, and it is not enough to draw a definite causal relationship. The sample size is also small, which may affect our analysis results. High-quality prospective multicenter studies are still needed for further analysis and confirmation in the future.

5. Conclusions

Under professional perioperative management, short-term preoperative discontinuation may help patients with antithrombotic therapy to obtain a relatively safe opportunity for TURP surgery. The risk of postoperative bleeding, VTE, and serious cardiovascular and cerebrovascular complications seems to be acceptable and controllable. It is essential for urologists to pay more attention to the perioperative management of these patients. However, this study is a single-center study with a small number of cases and thus needs further high-quality research results for more powerful verification.

Author Contributions: Methodology, Z.L., Z.Z., Q.Z. and Z.T.; Resources, Z.Z.; Data curation, Z.L., X.L., Q.Z., Z.W. and Z.T.; Writing—original draft, Z.L. and Z.W.; Writing—review & editing, Z.Z., K.L., L.H., Z.W. and Z.T. All authors have read and agreed to the published version of the manuscript.

Funding: This work was supported by the National Natural Science Foundation of China (82170706) and the Science and Technology Plan of the Department of Finance of Hunan Province (Hunan finance budget (2020) No. 09).

Institutional Review Board Statement: The study was conducted in accordance with the Declaration of Helsinki, and approved by the Ethics Committee of Xiangya Hospital of Central South University (No. 202011183).

Informed Consent Statement: Informed consent was obtained from all subjects involved in the study.

Data Availability Statement: Not applicable.

Conflicts of Interest: The authors declare that the research was conducted in the absence of any commercial or financial relationships that could be construed as a potential conflict of interest.

References

1. Rassweiler, J.; Teber, D.; Kuntz, R.; Hofmann, R. Complications of Transurethral Resection of the Prostate (TURP)—Incidence, Management, and Prevention. *Eur. Urol.* **2006**, *50*, 969–979, Discussion 80. [CrossRef] [PubMed]
2. Dornbier, R.; Pahouja, G.; Branch, J.; McVary, K.T. The New American Urological Association Benign Prostatic Hyperplasia Clinical Guidelines: 2019 Update. *Curr. Urol. Rep.* **2020**, *21*, 32. [CrossRef] [PubMed]
3. Mcvary, K.T.; Roehrborn, C.G.; Avins, A.L.; Barry, M.J.; Bruskewitz, R.C.; Donnell, R.F.; Foster, H.E., Jr.; Gonzalez, C.M.; Kaplan, S.A.; Penson, D.F.; et al. Update on AUA Guideline on the Management of Benign Prostatic Hyperplasia. *J. Urol.* **2011**, *185*, 1793–1803. [CrossRef] [PubMed]
4. Oelke, M.; Bachmann, A.; Descazeaud, A.; Emberton, M.; Gravas, S.; Michel, M.C.; N'Dow, J.; Nordling, J.; de la Rosette, J.J. EAU Guidelines on the Treatment and Follow-Up of Non-Neurogenic Male Lower Urinary Tract Symptoms Including Benign Prostatic Obstruction. *Eur. Urol.* **2013**, *64*, 118–140. [CrossRef]
5. Schulman, S.; Ageno, W.; Konstantinides, S.V. Venous Thromboembolism: Past, Present and Future. *Thromb. Haemost.* **2017**, *117*, 1219–1229. [CrossRef]
6. Decousus, H.; Quéré, I.; Presles, E.; Becker, F.; Barrellier, M.T.; Chanut, M.; Gillet, J.L.; Guenneguez, H.; Leandri, C.; Mismetti, P.; et al. Superficial Venous Thrombosis and Venous Thromboembolism: A Large, Prospective Epidemiologic Study. *Ann. Intern. Med.* **2010**, *152*, 218–224. [CrossRef]
7. Bauersachs, R.M.; Herold, J. Oral Anticoagulation in the Elderly and Frail. *Hamostaseologie* **2020**, *40*, 74–83. [CrossRef]
8. Shahar, E.; Folsom, A.R.; Room, F.J.; Bisgard, K.M.; Metcalf, P.A.; Crum, L.; McGovern, P.G.; Hutchinson, R.G.; Heiss, G. Patterns of Aspirin Use in Middle-Aged Adults: The Atherosclerosis Risk in Communities (ARIC) Study. *Am. Heart J.* **1996**, *131*, 915–922. [CrossRef]
9. Burger, W.; Chemnitius, J.M.; Kneissl, G.D.; Rücker, G. Low-Dose Aspirin for Secondary Cardiovascular Prevention—Cardiovascular Risks after Its Perioperative Withdrawal Versus Bleeding Risks with Its Continuation—Review And Meta-Analysis. *J. Intern. Med.* **2005**, *257*, 399–414. [CrossRef]

10. Wu, Z.Q.; Li, K.X.; Zhu, Q.; Li, H.Z.; Tang, Z.Y.; Wang, Z. Application Value of D-Dimer Testing and Caprini Risk Assessment Model (RAM) to Predict Venous Thromboembolism (VTE) in Chinese Non-Oncological Urological Inpatients: A Retrospective Study from a Tertiary Hospital. *Transl. Androl. Urol.* **2020**, *9*, 1904–1911. [CrossRef]
11. Giannarini, G.; Mogorovich, A.; Valent, F.; Morelli, G.; De Maria, M.; Manassero, F.; Barbone, F.; Selli, C. Continuing or Discontinuing Low-Dose Aspirin Before Transrectal Prostate Biopsy: Results of a Prospective Randomized Trial. *Urology* **2007**, *70*, 501–505. [CrossRef]
12. Dimitropoulos, K.; Omar, M.I.; Chalkias, A.; Arnaoutoglou, E.; Douketis, J.; Gravas, S. Perioperative Antithrombotic (Antiplatelet and Anticoagulant) Therapy in Urological Practice: A Critical Assessment and Summary of the Clinical Practice Guidelines. *World J. Urol.* **2020**, *38*, 2761–2770. [CrossRef] [PubMed]
13. Parikh, A.; Toepfer, N.; Baylor, K.; Henry, Y.; Berger, P.; Rukstalis, D. Preoperative Aspirin Is Safe in Patients Undergoing Urologic Robot-Assisted Surgery. *J. Endourol.* **2012**, *26*, 852–856. [CrossRef]
14. Ala-opas, M.Y.; Grönlund, S.S. Blood Loss in Long-Term Aspirin Users Undergoing Transurethral Prostatectomy. *Scand. J. Urol. Nephrol.* **1996**, *30*, 203–206. [CrossRef]
15. Herget, E.J.; Saliken, J.C.; Donnelly, B.J.; Gray, R.R.; Wiseman, D.; Brunet, G. Transrectal Ultrasound-Guided Biopsy Of The Prostate: Relation Between ASA Use And Bleeding Complications. *Can. Assoc. Radiol. J. J. L'association Can. Des Radiol.* **1999**, *50*, 173–176.
16. Afshari, A.; Ageno, W.; Ahmed, A.; Duranteau, J.; Faraoni, D.; Kozek-Langenecker, S.; Llau, J.; Nizard, J.; Solca, M.; Stensballe, J.; et al. European Guidelines on Perioperative Venous Thromboembolism Prophylaxis: Executive Summary. *Eur. J. Anaesthesiol.* **2018**, *35*, 77–83. [CrossRef]
17. Gu, F.L.; Xia, T.L.; Kong, X.T. Preliminary Study of The Frequency of Benign Prostatic Hyperplasia And Prostatic Cancer in China. *Urology* **1994**, *44*, 688–691. [CrossRef]
18. Lerner, L.B.; Mcvary, K.T.; Barry, M.J.; Bixler, B.R.; Dahm, P.; Das, A.K.; Gandhi, M.C.; Kaplan, S.A.; Kohler, T.S.; Martin, L.; et al. Management of Lower Urinary Tract Symptoms Attributed to Benign Prostatic Hyperplasia: AUA GUIDELINE PART II-Surgical Evaluation And Treatment. *J. Urol.* **2021**, *206*, 818–826. [CrossRef]
19. Go, A.S.; Hylek, E.M.; Phillips, K.A.; Chang, Y.; Henault, L.E.; Selby, J.V.; Singer, D.E. Prevalence of Diagnosed Atrial Fibrillation in Adults: National Implications for Rhythm Management and Stroke Prevention: The Anticoagulation and Risk Factors in Atrial Fibrillation (ATRIA) Study. *JAMA* **2001**, *285*, 2370–2375. [CrossRef]
20. Lebdai, S.; Robert, G.; Devonnec, M.; Fourmarier, M.; Haillot, O.; Saussine, C.; Azzouzi, A.R.; De La Taille, A.; Descazeaud, A. Management of Patients under Anticoagulants for Transurethral Resection of the Prostate: A Multicentric Study by the CTMH-AFU. *Prog. En Urol. J. De L'association Fr. D'urologie Et De La Soc. Fr. D'urologie* **2009**, *19*, 553–557. [CrossRef]
21. Wendt-Nordahl, G.; Bucher, B.; Häcker, A.; Knoll, T.; Alken, P.; Michel, M.S. Improvement in Mortality and Morbidity in Transurethral Resection of the Prostate over 17 Years in A Single Center. *J. Endourol.* **2007**, *21*, 1081–1087. [CrossRef] [PubMed]
22. Uchida, T.; Ohori, M.; Soh, S.; Sato, T.; Iwamura, M.; Ao, T.; Koshiba, K. Factors Influencing Morbidity in Patients Undergoing Transurethral Resection of the Prostate. *Urology* **1999**, *53*, 98–105. [CrossRef] [PubMed]
23. Reich, O.; Gratzke, C.; Bachmann, A.; Seitz, M.; Schlenker, B.; Hermanek, P.; Lack, N.; Stief, C.G. Morbidity, Mortality And Early Outcome of Transurethral Resection of the Prostate: A Prospective Multicenter Evaluation of 10,654 Patients. *J. Urol.* **2008**, *180*, 246–249. [CrossRef] [PubMed]
24. Taylor, K.; Filgate, R.; Guo, D.Y.; Macneil, F. A Retrospective Study to Assess the Morbidity Associated with Transurethral Prostatectomy in Patients on Antiplatelet or Anticoagulant Drugs. *BJU Int.* **2011**, *108*, 45–50. [CrossRef]
25. Tikkinen, K.; Cartwright, R.; Gould, M.; Naspro, R.; Novara, G.; Sandset, P.; Violette, P.; Guyatt, G. EAU Guidelines on Thromboprophylaxis in Urological Surgery. In Proceedings of the 32nd EAU Annual Meeting, London, UK, 24–28 March 2017.
26. Mcquaid, K.R.; Laine, L. Systematic Review and Meta-Analysis of Adverse Events of Low-Dose Aspirin and Clopidogrel in Randomized Controlled Trials. *Am. J. Med.* **2006**, *119*, 624–638. [CrossRef]
27. Wierød, F.S.; Frandsen, N.J.; Jacobsen, J.D.; Hartvigsen, A.; Olsen, P.R. Risk of Haemorrhage from Transurethral Prostatectomy in Acetylsalicylic Acid and NSAID-Treated Patients. *Scand. J. Urol. Nephrol.* **1998**, *32*, 120–122.
28. Zhu, J.P.; Davidsen, M.B.; Meyhoff, H.H. Aspirin, A Silent Risk Factor in Urology. *Scand. J. Urol. Nephrol.* **1995**, *29*, 369–374. [CrossRef]
29. Allaway, M.G.R.; Eslick, G.D.; Kwok, G.T.Y.; Cox, M.R. Improving Venous Thromboembolism Prophylaxis Administration in an Acute Surgical Unit. *J. Patient Saf.* **2021**, *17*, E1341–E1345. [CrossRef]
30. Golash, A.; Collins, P.W.; Kynaston, H.G.; Jenkins, B.J. Venous Thromboembolic Prophylaxis for Transurethral Prostatectomy: Practice Among British Urologists. *J. R. Soc. Med.* **2002**, *95*, 130–131. [CrossRef]
31. Mcalpine, K.; Breau, R.H.; Mallick, R.; Cnossen, S.; Cagiannos, I.; Morash, C.; Carrier, M.; Lavallée, L.T. Current Guidelines Do Not Sufficiently Discriminate Venous Thromboembolism Risk in Urology. *Urol. Oncol.* **2017**, *35*, 457.e1–457.e8. [CrossRef]
32. Marchiori, A.; Mosena, L.; Prandoni, P. Superficial Vein Thrombosis: Risk Factors, Diagnosis, And Treatment. *Semin. Thromb. Hemost.* **2006**, *32*, 737–743. [CrossRef]

33. Shaw, N.M.; Hakam, N.; Lui, J.L.; Nabavizadeh, B.; Li, K.D.; Low, P.; Abbasi, B.; Breyer, B.N. Incidence of Venous Thromboembolism in Benign Urologic Reconstructive Cases. *World J. Urol.* **2022**, *40*, 1879–1886. [CrossRef] [PubMed]
34. Li, K.; Zhu, Q.; Li, H.; Wu, Z.; Han, F.; Tang, Z.; Wang, Z. Incidence, Risk Factors, Risk Assessment Model and Compliance of Patients on Anticoagulants for Asymptomatic Venous Thromboembolism in Nononcological Urological Inpatients. *Urol. J.* **2021**, *20*, 56–65.

Disclaimer/Publisher's Note: The statements, opinions and data contained in all publications are solely those of the individual author(s) and contributor(s) and not of MDPI and/or the editor(s). MDPI and/or the editor(s) disclaim responsibility for any injury to people or property resulting from any ideas, methods, instructions or products referred to in the content.

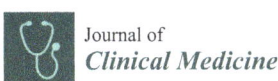

Article

Laser Efficiency and Laser Safety: Holmium YAG vs. Thulium Fiber Laser

Alba Sierra [1,2,3], Mariela Corrales [2,3], Bhaskar Somani [4] and Olivier Traxer [2,3,*]

1. Urology Department, Hospital Clínic de Barcelona, Villarroel 170, 08036 Barcelona, Spain
2. GRC Urolithiasis No. 20, Tenon Hospital, Sorbonne University, F-75020 Paris, France
3. Department of Urology AP-HP, Tenon Hospital, Sorbonne University, F-75020 Paris, France
4. Urology Department, University Hospital Southampton NHS Trust, Southampton SO16 6YD, UK
* Correspondence: olivier.traxer@aphp.fr

Abstract: (1) Objective: To support the efficacy and safety of a range of thulium fiber laser (TFL) pre-set parameters for laser lithotripsy: the efficiency is compared against the Holmium:YAG (Ho:YAG) laser in the hands of juniors and experienced urologists using an in vitro ureteral model; the ureteral damage of both lasers is evaluated in an in vivo porcine model. (2) Materials and Methods: Ho:YAG laser technology and TFL technology, with a 200 μm core-diameter laser fibers in an in vitro saline ureteral model were used. Each participant performed 12 laser sessions. Each session included a 3-min lasering of stone phantoms (Begostone) with each laser technology in six different pre-settings retained from the Coloplast TFL Drive user interface pre-settings, for stone dusting: 0.5 J/10 Hz, 0.5 J/20 Hz, 0.7 J/10 Hz, 0.7 J/20 Hz, 1 J/12 Hz and 1 J/20 Hz. Both lasers were also used in three in vivo porcine models, lasering up to 20 W and 12 W in the renal pelvis and the ureter, respectively. Temperature was continuously recorded. After 3 weeks, a second look was done to verify the integrity of the ureters and kidney and an anatomopathological analysis was performed. (3) Results: Regarding laser lithotripsy efficiency, after 3 min of continuous lasering, the overall ablation rate (AR) percentage was 27% greater with the TFL technology ($p < 0.0001$). The energy per ablated mass [J/mg] was 24% lower when using the TFL ($p < 0.0001$). While junior urologists performed worse than seniors in all tests, they performed better when using the TFL than Ho:YAG technology (36% more AR and 36% fewer J/mg). In the in vivo porcine model, no urothelial damage was observed for both laser technologies, neither endoscopically during lasering, three weeks later, nor in the pathological test. (4) Conclusions: By using Coloplast TFL Drive GUI pre-set, TFL lithotripsy efficiency is higher than Ho:YAG laser, even in unexperienced hands. Concerning urothelial damage, both laser technologies with low power present no lesions.

Keywords: holmium YAG; thulium fiber laser; lithotripsy; laser settings; laser efficiency; laser safety; laser usability; kidney calculi; ureteroscopy

1. Introduction

Ureteroscopy with laser lithotripsy is an extended surgical intervention used for urinary stone treatment [1]. The current gold standard laser is the Holmium YAG (Ho:YAG) laser. One of the latest technologies in laser lithotripsy is the thulium fiber laser (TFL) which uses a 10–20 μm silica fiber doped with elemental thulium to generate the laser beam. When compared to Ho:YAG technology, TFL technology results are more efficient, with an ablation rate of up to three times higher and a retropulsion value that is about three times lower [2–4]. Despite the consistent technological improvement in this field, there is a lack of consensus regarding the parameters to use [5] and a need for high-level evidence when it comes to TFL vs. Ho:YAG [6,7].

On the other hand, one of the major concerns with this new technology is its safety. Some authors believe that the more efficient absorption in water (1.9 μm for TFL and

2.1 µm for Ho:YAG) [8] may lead to more pronounced heating of the aqueous environment, causing indirect urothelial thermal injury [9–11]. To manage the double issue of safety management and choice of effective parameters, pre-settings might be helpful.

The aim of this study was to evaluate the relevance of low-power settings to manage effective stone dusting while maintaining safety during TFL lithotripsy. To test laser lithotripsy efficiency, a range of pre-settings as retained by Coloplast TFL Drive interface for stone dusting is compared between the holmium:YAG (Ho:YAG) laser and thulium fiber laser (TFL) in the hands of juniors and experienced urologists, using an in vitro ureteral model. Urothelial damage of both lasers was evaluated in an in vivo porcine model.

2. Materials and Methods

2.1. Laser Lithotripsy Efficiency

2.1.1. Laser Systems

The Cyber: Ho 150 WTM (Ho:YAG laser) and the Fiber Dust (TFL) were used as laser generators. Both lasers were from Quanta System (Samarate, Lombardia, Italy). We chose those devices because the laser settings can be set identically in both laser generators (pulse energy and frequency).

2.1.2. Artificial Stones

We produced stone phantoms (5 mm cubes) according to previously described techniques [12]. Matching Begostone Plus powder (Bego France®, Villeurbanne, France) with distilled water, we aimed to reproduce calcium–oxalate monohydrate stones. A «powder to water» ratio of 15:3 was chosen, according to previous in vitro studies [13]. After confection, a drying period of 48 h at 30 °C was maintained to minimize the heterogeneity between stones. All stones were weighed with a digital balance (ASP-22E-001 Analytic Balance RADWAG serie) with 0.001 mg accuracy after the drying period.

2.1.3. Experimental Setup

The custom experimental setting, as previously described by [3], consisted of a ureteral model (polymer tube 17 cm length, closed on one side, 7 mm inner diameter), with an opaque tape on a tray with saline (Figure 1).

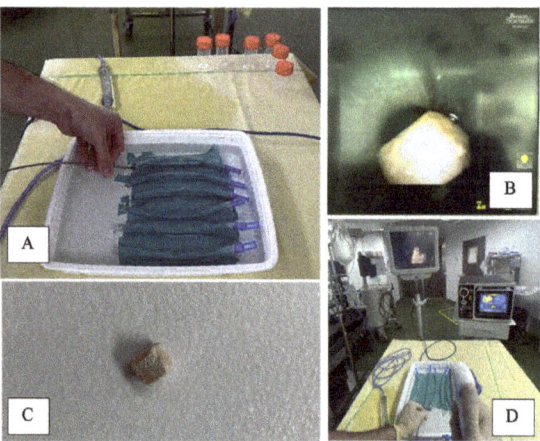

Figure 1. Experimental set up showing (**A**) Six polymer tubes, 17 cm length, closed on one side, 7 mm diameter, with an opaque tape on a tray with saline, used as a ureteral model (**B**) Endovision of the ureteral model with a Lithovue (Boston Scientific®, Maple Grove, MN, USA) and a BegoStone on it (**C**) BegoStone 5 × 5 × 5 mm^3, dry weigh before and after the tests (**D**) Room display, using a Lithovue (Boston Scientific®, Maple Grove, MN, USA). Irrigation was ensured by a combination of a gravity irrigation at 40 cmH$_2$O above the saline tray and a hand-assisted irrigation system.

Trials were conducted using a single use digital flexible ureteroscope (Lithovue, Boston Scientific©, Maple Grove, MN, USA). Irrigation was ensured by a combination of a gravity irrigation at 40 cmH$_2$O above the saline tray and a hand-assisted irrigation system providing on-demand forced irrigation to offer proper visibility, as is done in routine clinical practice (Figure 1).

Participants were divided into two groups according to their skills (five junior urologists and five senior urologists performing more than 80 URS per year). Each one performed 12 continuous lasering sessions (6 with TFL and 6 with Ho:YAG laser) of 3 min with the following laser settings retained from the user interface pre-settings of the Coloplast TFL Drive for stone dusting: 0.5 J/10 Hz, 0.5 J/20 Hz, 0.7 J/10 Hz, 0.7 J/20 Hz, 1 J/12 Hz, 1 J/20 Hz. All tests were performed with a short pulse width from the manufacturer's laser console settings and a 200 µm core-diameter silica fiber.

Data included laser settings (energy and frequency) and total energy. All stone fragments were labeled and dried at room temperature (21 °C).

2.1.4. Statistical Analysis

SPSS v25 software (IBM Statistics, Chicago, IL, USA) was used for the statistical analysis. Ablation rates of different laser settings and equipment were recorded and analyzed. For each cohort of laser generators and set of laser parameters, 12 trials were performed. Results are presented as mean and percentages. To assess laser efficiency, one way ANOVA and T-student tests were used. A p-value of 0.05 or less was considered significant.

2.2. Urothelial Damage

2.2.1. Experimental Setup

Studies adhered to the Guide for the Care and Use of Laboratory Animals under an approval of Regional Animal Ethical Committee (#CEEA14). A French Government authorization and were conducted at CERC Faculté de Médecine Nord, Marseille, France (IACUC) (#D-13-055-22).

Three female pigs were used for the experimentation (~40 kg). All procedures were performed under general anesthesia. The anesthetized pigs were placed in the dorsal position. A rigid cystoscopy was used to place a 0.035" guidewire (Terumo, Tokyo, Japan) into the pig kidney, and then a ureteral access sheath (UAS, Retrace 12/14 Fh, Coloplast, Denmark) was placed. A flexible ureteroscope was then positioned in the renal pelvis. An endoscopic evaluation of the renal pelvis was performed (Figure 2). We started the lasering in the renal pelvis, and then, in the distal ureter (after UAS removal), without touching the mucosa.

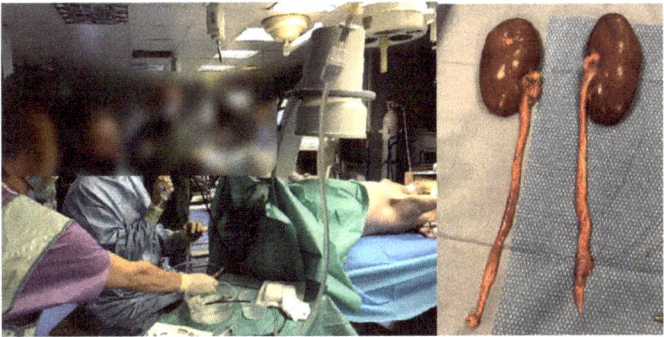

Figure 2. Female pigs (~40 kg). All procedures were performed under general anesthesia and the pigs were placed in the dorsal position. After the first procedure, pigs were kept alive and a second ureteroscopy was performed 18 days later to check for endoscopically tissue lesions. Animals were then sacrificed, and organs were removed for anatomopathological analysis.

2.2.2. Laser Settings

The Cyber: Ho 150 WTM and the Fiber Dust generators (Quanta System Samarate, Lombardia, Italy) were used. Power limits were 20 W (1 J/20 Hz) and 12 W (1 J/12 Hz) in the kidney and ureter, respectively. All tests were performed with short pulse width and a 200 µm core-diameter silica fiber. In all pigs, TFL was used in the left ureter/kidney and Ho:YAG was used in the right ureter/kidney. We performed continuous lasering in the renal pelvis and in the renal papilla for 10 min in each area, to simulate the worst-case scenario. Then, we performed the same technique for 7 min (half on/half off) at the middle of the lumen of the proximal and distal ureter. Continuous irrigation was established at 40 cmH$_2$O.

2.2.3. Method of Temperature Measurement

Before lasering, temperature was continuously recorded by a probe wire retrogradely inserted in the renal cavities that transmitted the intrarenal temperature into a console in the third pig.

2.2.4. Post-Procedure Endoscopic Control

Urothelial injuries heal 5–10 days after their formation. To check tissue healing lesions, pigs were kept alive until a second ureteroscopy 18 days later. An endoscopic diagnosis exploration was made, and their kidneys and ureters were sent for analysis (Figure 2). Pathological analysis was performed by an independent laboratory to assess healing/fibrotic process.

3. Results

3.1. Laser Efficiency

After 3 min of continue lasering, the overall ablation rate (AR) percentage of Begostone was 27% ($p < 0.0001$) greater with the TFL than with the Ho:YAG technology (Table 1). When comparing each setting, the overall mean AR was also superior for all groups using the TFL technology. Despite the laser source, differences were also found regarding AR ($p < 0.001$); the more delivered energy, the higher the AR. Similar results were found when comparing energy per stone weight (J/mg). The overall J/mg was 24% ($p < 0.0001$) lower when using the TFL than the Ho:YAG (Table 2) lasers.

Table 1. Ablation rate (mg/s) of each scenario by Ho:YAG and TFL lasers, during 3 min of laser lithotripsy. Holmium YAG (Ho:YAG). Thulium fiber laser (TFL).

			Laser Settings							Ureter Tested Settings	All Tested Settings
			0.5 J/10 Hz *	0.5 J/20 Hz *	0.7 J/10 Hz *	0.7 J/20 Hz *	1 J/12 Hz *	1 J/20 Hz		
			Ablation rate (mg/s)								
Junior (n = 5)	Mean	Ho:YAG	8.24	10.04	17.12	28.18	41.26	41.44	19.165	24.38
		TFL	13.28	17.52	22.7	38.04	50.96	56.82	26.115	33.22
	% Difference		−52%	+61%	+74%	+32%	+35%	+23%	+37%	+36%
	p value		0.10	0.1	0.03	<0.001	<0.0001	<0.001	<0.001	<0.0001
Senior (n = 5)	Mean	Ho:YAG	19.58	28.4	22.5	46.52	49.92	61.34	30.1	38.04
		TFL	26.08	31.2	30.44	59	58.56	70.82	36.57	46.02
	% Difference		−19%	+33%	+10%	+35%	+27%	+17%	+15%	+21%
	p value		0.04	0.02	0.15	<0.0001	0.004	0.0001	<0.0001	<0.0001
Total group (n = 10)	Mean	Ho:YAG	13.91	19.22	19.81	37.35	45.59	51.39	24.63	31.21
		TFL	19.68	24.36	26.57	48.52	54.76	63.82	31.34	39.62
	% Difference		−33%	+41%	+27%	+34%	+30%	+20%	+24%	+27%
	p value		0.002	0.008	<0.0001	<0.0001	<0.0001	<0.0001	<0.0001	<0.0001

* Coloplast TFL Drive user interface pre-settings for stone dusting in the ureter (≤12 W). Red front color means statistical significancy because is < 0.05.

Table 2. Comparison thulium fiber laser vs Holmium:YAG. Energy/stone weight (J/mg) in each scenario after 3 min of laser lithotripsy. Holmium YAG (Ho:YAG). Thulium fiber laser (TFL).

			Laser Settings						Ureter Tested Settings	All Tested Settings
			0.5 J/10 Hz *	0.5 J/20 Hz *	0.7 J/10 Hz *	0.7 J/20 Hz	1 J/12 Hz *	1 J/20 Hz		
			Energy/stone volume (J/mg)							
Junior (n = 5)	Mean	Ho:YAG	21.07	29.64	14.21	16.52	8.71	14.97	19.04	17.52
		TFL	10.03	19.25	10.26	10.11	7.25	10.48	13.34	11.23
	% Difference		−52%	−35%	−28%	−39%	−17%	−30%	−70%	−36%
	p value		0.10	0.13	0.002	<0.0001	0.24	0.001	0.002	<0.0001
Senior (n = 5)	Mean	Ho:YAG	8.05	7.87	9.12	8.93	6.73	9.07	8.21	8.30
		TFL	6.52	10.63	7.82	6.68	7.08	7.14	8.21	7.64
	% Difference		−19%	+35%	−14%	−25%	+5%	−21%	0%	−19%
	p value		0.04	0.02	0.05	0.06	0.77	0.04	0.99	0.07
Total group (n = 10)	Mean	Ho:YAG	14.77	19.04	12.61	13.29	8.06	12.31	13.62	13.35
		TFL	9.95	16.14	9.63	8.66	7.38	8.94	10.78	10.12
	% Difference		−33%	−15%	−24%	−35%	−8%	−27%	−21%	−24%
	p value		0.06	0.17	0.0008	0.0002	0.32	0.001	0.004	<0.0001

* Coloplast TFL Drive user interface pre-settings for stone dusting in the ureter (≤12 W). Red front color means statistical significancy because is <0.05.

When comparing per expertise, junior urologists performed worse than seniors in all the tests for both lasers, AR percentage and energy per stone weight, but both juniors and seniors performed better when using TFL technology. However, when comparing their performance using TFL versus Ho:YAG lasers, juniors improved more than seniors (15% more AR percentage and 17% less J/mg).

For ureteral stone treatment, the recommended laser power setting is less than 12 W [14]. Suggested settings for ureteral stones have 24% ($p < 0.0001$) better AR percentage and 21% ($p = 0.004$) lower energy per weight (J/mg) with TFL technology.

3.2. Urothelial Damage

Left and right urinary tracts were treated by TFL and Ho:YAG, respectively. A total of 23 tests were performed using three female pigs. The four defined sites were the renal papilla, renal pelvis and proximal and distal ureter. Due to time constraints, the left distal ureter of the third pig could not be tested.

First evaluation was performed endoscopically during laser activation. After 10 min of continuous lasering in the renal pelvis and the papilla, some small hyperemic lesions were seen in all kidneys with both Ho:YAG and TFL with no subjective differences between lasers using same power settings (Figure 3). No lesions were observed after seven sequential minutes (half on/half off) in the ureter for both lasers. Moreover, the maximal powers used (12 W and 20 W for ureter and kidney, respectively) were not accompanied with per-procedure safety issues. There was no bleeding, no perforation and no carbonization.

During the third pig's laser lithotripsy, the temperature was continuously recorded. In the left kidney (TFL), the temperature increased from 31.5 °C to 36.8 °C after 1.5 min of lasering. For 3 min, we progressively decreased irrigation until it stopped completely reaching a maximum of 40.2 °C. With continuous irrigation, the temperature remained around 36 °C during lasering and decreased below 35 °C when lasering stopped. For the right kidney (Ho:YAG), the temperature quickly increased from 33 °C to 41 °C when irrigation was slowed down until it stopped completely and remained between 33 °C and 34.6 °C during irrigation.

The second evaluation was performed endoscopically three weeks after laser lithotripsy. To access the renal pelvis, a UAS was inserted. Unspecific white marks were found in all kidneys, located at the upper papilla or peri-papilla and the renal pelvis (Figure 3). After

UAS removal, ureteral evaluation was performed, and no lesions were found in neither the proximal nor distal ureter. Of note, in the third pig, where the temperature test was performed and the irrigation was voluntarily reduced, Bellini tubules were visible in both kidneys.

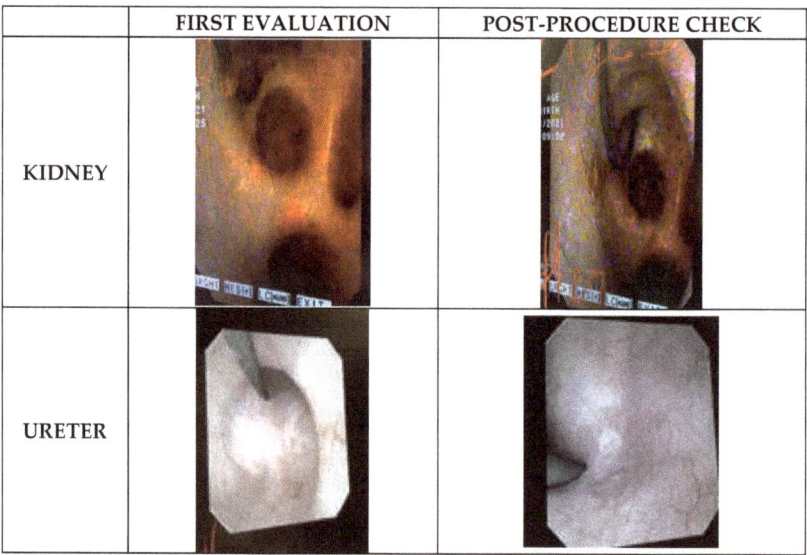

Figure 3. Endoscopic images captured during first evaluation and three weeks later, for kidney and ureter sites. Subjectively no differences were found endoscopically between TFL and Ho:YAG during per-procedure and post-procedure safety check.

No differences were detected after anatomopathological evaluation for both lasers and only slight inflammation was seen in some cases. Regarding the renal parenchyma, all animals had interstitial nephritis on both kidneys and showed no differences between Ho:YAG and TFL.

4. Discussion

According to our results, TFL technology is superior to the Ho:YAG laser with better AR. This is not the first time that the TFL had performed better than the Ho:YAG laser [2,3,8]. Preclinical studies have shown promising results with a more efficient stone ablation rate and a faster ablation speed with TFL [8]. At the same energy and pulse frequency settings, TFL technology produces a significantly lower retropulsion rate than the current Ho:YAG technology [4]. This can be explained by several of the TFL's characteristics. For instance, the fourfold higher wavelength absorption by water may result in greater absorption of laser energy during laser lithotripsy and also explain its high ablation efficiency over any type of stone [15–17]. Additionally, when focusing on peak power and pulse shape, the Ho:YAG's peak power is extremely variable. On the contrary, TFL exhibits a nearly rectangular flat-top pulse shape with an almost constant low peak power (500 W) at different settings. At equivalent energy settings, the pulse generated by the TFL in SP mode is longer and has a lower peak power than the one of the Ho:YAG laser in the long pulse and Moses pulse modes [4,15]. These characteristics have been confirmed in several clinical studies after the approval of the US Food and Drug Administration and European CE mark in 2019 and 2020, respectively [6,18]. Even if clinical experiences are still low, we are starting to see high-quality trials with this new technology. Ulvik et al. [7] have recently published the first prospective randomized trial, showing that the TFL is superior to the Ho:YAG laser in terms of the stone-free rate, shorter operative time and fewer intraoperative complications.

In addition, TFL seems to be more worthwhile for learners. When comparing results based on expertise, junior urologists performed worse than experienced urologist in all tests for both AR percentage and energy/stone weight. However, despite that, juniors performed better when using TFL technology, showing a reduced learning curve and lack of need to constantly adapt to a continuously changing stone position. This can be explained by the lower degree of retropulsion with TFL, which helps to improve the precision and vision during stone ablation [19]. Several lab studies have shown that TFL has lower retropulsion than Ho:YAG laser [4,18,20], leading to a more efficient lithotripsy [21]. Several clinical trials have also shown that TFL is a safe and effective modality for laser lithotripsy because of the lower retropulsion and minimal complication rate [22–25].

Although Ho:YAG has demonstrate an excellent safety profile, being considered as the more successful laser, TFL wavelength (1940 nm) is closer to water absorption peak, which results in four-fold higher abortion than Ho:YAG. This facilitates higher absorption of energy and increased ablation efficiency [8]. However, this higher rate of energy transfer to the stone and the surrounding fluid could potentially lead to indirect thermal damage [9–11]. Recently, Belle JD et al. [11] have demonstrated, in an in vitro silicone kidney-ureter model, that high-power lasers are associated with a risk of complications from thermal damage and therefore advocate using rather conservative laser settings for ureteroscopy laser lithotripsy. According to previously published papers, temperature rises proportionally to power [25], and power limits are settled at 20–30 W and 10–15 W for the kidney and ureter, respectively, to avoid cellular thermal damage [3,9,10]. Our study results are in line with that statement. We remark that low power settings are safe for the urothelium, as we confirmed in our second look of the porcine kidney. Moreover, the use of saline irrigation during the procedure has shown to be critical to avoid excessive temperature rises, and studies evaluating temperature rise with both Ho:YAG and TFL have demonstrated a good safety profile when continuous irrigation was applied during laser activation [10,26,27]. Similar findings are described during our trial, we were continuously lasering with continuous irrigation at 40 cmH$_2$O and temperature remained at 36.8 °C and 34.6 °C for TFL and Ho:YAG, respectively.

Regarding laser effectivity, we tried to simulate a real-life scenario, but the first limitation was an incomplete simulation of actual laser lithotripsy conditions in a urinary tract. Such conditions included ureteral peristalsis, respiratory movements and convection, which plays major roles during laser lithotripsy in the ureter. However, the aim of our study was to compare different settings and the obtained ablation rate. Stone phantoms, rather than human stones, were used. We required samples of approximately uniform mass, geometry, and composition, which could not be achieved practically with human stones. The third limitation involved the BegoStones immediately absorbing water through cracks and pores, which would have influenced the results of dehydrated phantoms in water. It should also be mentioned that the so-called dry phantoms in our study had not been desiccated. However, we have a control stone that was submerged into the saline tray without lithotripsy treatment, and we stored the stones in similar conditions. When its weight was the same as before the experiment, we assumed that the rest were dried too. In the porcine model, we were not lasering to stones, but we simulated the worst-case scenario through 10 min continuous lasering in the same place.

5. Conclusions

In vitro, laser lithotripsy efficiency is higher with the TFL than with the Ho:YAG laser. Indeed, despite low power settings, AR was significantly higher, and less energy was needed to ablate 1 mg of stone with the TFL. Interestingly, it seemed that junior urologists had a faster learning curve with the TFL than with the Ho:YAG laser. Concerning laser safety, both laser technologies are equally safe. We can conclude than the Coloplast TFL Drive GUI pre-set values are effective and safe when working with 20 W in the kidney and 12 W in the ureter.

Author Contributions: Conceptualization, A.S. and M.C.; methodology, O.T.; formal analysis, M.C.; investigation, A.S., M.C. and O.T.; original draft preparation, A.S.; writing—review and editing, A.S. and B.S.; supervision, O.T. All authors have read and agreed to the published version of the manuscript.

Funding: This research received no external funding.

Institutional Review Board Statement: The study was conducted according to the guidelines of the Declaration of Helsinki, and adhered to the Guide for the Care and Use of Laboratory Animals under an approved Institutional Animal Care and Use Committee (IACUC) protocol (#D-13-055-22).

Informed Consent Statement: Not applicable.

Data Availability Statement: Ask to the authors.

Conflicts of Interest: Alba Sierra and Mariela Corrales have nothing to disclose. Olivier Traxer is a consultant for Boston Scientific, Coloplast, EMS, IPG, Quanta and Rocamed, but has no specific conflicts relevant to this work.

References

1. Geraghty, R.M.; Davis, N.F.; Tzelves, L.; Lombardo, R.; Yuan, C.; Thomas, K.; Petrik, A.; Neisius, A.; Türk, C.; Gambaro, G.; et al. Best Practice in Interventional Management of Urolithiasis: An Update from the European Association of Urology Guidelines Panel for Urolithiasis 2022. *Eur. Urol. Focus* **2022**. [CrossRef] [PubMed]
2. Andreeva, V.; Vinarov, A.; Yaroslavsky, I.; Kovalenko, A.; Vybornov, A.; Rapoport, L.; Enikeev, D.; Sorokin, N.; Dymov, A.; Tsarichenko, D.; et al. Preclinical comparison of superpulse thulium fiber laser and a holmium: YAG laser for lithotripsy. *World J. Urol.* **2020**, *38*, 497–503. [CrossRef] [PubMed]
3. Del Rio, A.S.; Corrales, M.; Kolvatzis, M.; Panthier, F.; Piñero, A.; Traxer, O. Thermal injury and laser efficiency with holmium: Yag and thulium fiber laser—An in vitro study. *J. Endourol.* **2022**, *36*, 1599–1606. [CrossRef]
4. Ventimiglia, E.; Doizi, S.; Kovalenko, A.; Andreeva, V.; Traxer, O. Effect of temporal pulse shape on urinary stone phantom retropulsion rate and ablation efficiency using holmium:YAG and super-pulse thulium fibre lasers. *BJU Int.* **2020**, *126*, 159–167. [CrossRef]
5. Sierra, A.; Corrales, M.; Piñero, A.; Traxer, O. Thulium fiber laser pre-settings during ureterorenoscopy: Twitter's experts' recommendations. *World J. Urol.* **2022**, *40*, 1529–1535. [CrossRef]
6. Traxer, O.; Corrales, M. Managing Urolithiasis with Thulium Fiber Laser: Updated Real-Life Results—A Systematic Review. *J. Clin. Med.* **2021**, *10*, 3390. [CrossRef]
7. Ulvik, Ø.; Æsøy, M.S.; Juliebø-Jones, P.; Gjengstø, P.; Beisland, C. Thulium Fibre Laser versus Holmium:YAG for Ureteroscopic Lithotripsy: Outcomes from a Prospective Randomised Clinical Trial. *Eur. Urol.* **2022**, *82*, 73–79. [CrossRef]
8. Kronenberg, P.; Traxer, O. The laser of the future: Reality and expectations about the new thulium fiber laser—A systematic review. *Transl. Androl. Urol.* **2019**, *8* (Suppl. 4), S398–S417. [CrossRef]
9. Taratkin, M.; Laukhtina, E.; Singla, N.; Kozlov, V.; Abdusalamov, A.; Ali, S.; Gabdullina, S.; Alekseeva, T.; Enikeev, D. Temperature changes during laser lithotripsy with Ho:YAG laser and novel Tm-fiber laser: A comparative in-vitro study. *World J. Urol.* **2020**, *38*, 3261–3266. [CrossRef]
10. Molina, W.R.; Carrera, R.V.; Chew, B.H.; Knudsen, B.E. Temperature rise during ureteral laser lithotripsy: Comparison of super pulse thulium fiber laser (SPTF) vs high power 120 W holmium-YAG laser (Ho:YAG). *World J. Urol.* **2021**, *39*, 3951–3956. [CrossRef]
11. Belle, J.D.; Chen, R.; Srikureja, N.; Amasyali, A.S.; Keheila, M.; Baldwin, D.D. Does the Novel Thulium Fiber Laser Have a Higher Risk of Urothelial Thermal Injury than the Conventional Holmium Laser in an In Vitro Study? *J. Endourol.* **2022**, *36*, 1249–1254. [CrossRef]
12. Esch, E.; Simmons, W.N.; Sankin, G.; Cocks, H.F.; Preminger, G.M.; Zhong, P. A simple method for fabricating artificial kidney stones of different physical properties. *Urol. Res.* **2010**, *38*, 315–319. [CrossRef] [PubMed]
13. Panthier, F.; Germain, T.; Gorny, C.; Berthe, L.; Doizi, S.; Traxer, O. Laser Fiber Displacement Velocity during Tm-Fiber and Ho:YAG Laser lithotripsy: Introducing the Concept of Optimal Displacement Velocity. *J. Clin. Med.* **2021**, *11*, 181. [CrossRef] [PubMed]
14. Sierra, A.; Corrales, M.; Kolvatzis, M.; Traxer, O. Initial clinical experience with the thulium fiber laser from Quanta System: First 50 reported cases. *World J. Urol.* **2022**, *40*, 2549–2553. [CrossRef] [PubMed]
15. Ventimiglia, E.; Villa, L.; Doizi, S.; Briganti, A.; Proietti, S.; Giusti, G.; Montorsi, F.; Montanari, E.; Traxer, O.; Salonia, A. Laser lithotripsy: The importance of peak power and pulse modulation. *Eur. Urol. Focus* **2021**, *7*, 22–25. [CrossRef]
16. Taratkin, M.; Laukhtina, E.; Singla, N.; Tarasov, A.; Alekseeva, T.; Enikeev, M.; Enikeev, D. How Lasers Ablate Stones: In Vitro Study of Laser Lithotripsy (Ho:YAG and Tm-Fiber Lasers) in Different Environments. *J. Endourol.* **2021**, *35*, 931–936. [CrossRef] [PubMed]
17. Keller, E.X.; De Coninck, V.; Doizi, S.; Daudon, M.; Traxer, O. Thulium fiber laser: Ready to dust all urinary stone composition types? *World J. Urol.* **2020**, *39*, 1693–1698. [CrossRef]

18. Kronenberg, P.; Hameed, B.Z.; Somani, B. Outcomes of thulium fibre laser for treatment of urinary tract stones: Results of a systematic review. *Curr. Opin. Urol.* **2021**, *31*, 80–86. [CrossRef] [PubMed]
19. Miller, C.S.; Whiles, B.B.; Ito, W.E.; Machen, E.; Thompson, J.A.; Duchene, D.A.; Neff, D.A.; Molina, W.R. Image Distortion During Flexible Ureteroscopy: A Laboratory Model Comparing SuperPulsed Thulium Fiber Laser vs. High-Power Ho:YAG Laser. *J. Endourol.* **2022**. [CrossRef]
20. Enikeev, D.; Shariat, S.F.; Taratkin, M.; Glybochko, P. The changing role of lasers in urologic surgery. *Curr. Opin. Urol.* **2020**, *30*, 24–29. [CrossRef]
21. Gao, B.; Bobrowski, A.; Lee, J. A scoping review of the clinical efficacy and safety of the novel thulium fiber laser: The rising star of laser lithotripsy. *Can. Urol. Assoc. J.* **2020**, *15*, 56–66. [CrossRef] [PubMed]
22. Martov, A.; Ergakov, D.; Guseynov, M.; Coninck, V.; Keller, E.; Traxer, O. VS1-2 SuperPulse Thulium Fiber Laser for Ureteroscopic Lithotripsy: 1 Year Experience. *J. Endourol.* **2018**, *32*, A495.
23. Korolev, D.; Akopyan, G.; Tsarichenko, D.; Shpikina, A.; Ali, S.; Chinenov, D.; Corrales, M.; Taratkin, M.; Traxer, O.; Enikeev, D. Minimally invasive percutaneous nephrolithotomy with SuperPulsed Thulium-fiber laser. *Urolithiasis* **2021**, *49*, 485–491. [CrossRef] [PubMed]
24. Enikeev, D.; Taratkin, M.; Klimov, R.; Alyaev, Y.; Rapoport, L.; Gazimiev, M.; Korolev, D.; Ali, S.; Akopyan, G.; Tsarichenko, D.; et al. Thulium-fiber laser for lithotripsy: First clinical experience in percutaneous nephrolithotomy. *World J. Urol.* **2020**, *38*, 3069–3074. [CrossRef] [PubMed]
25. De Coninck, V.; Defraigne, C.; Traxer, O. Watt determines the temperature during laser lithotripsy. *World J. Urol.* **2022**, *40*, 1257–1258. [CrossRef] [PubMed]
26. Wollin, D.A.; Carlos, E.C.; Tom, W.R.; Simmons, W.N.; Preminger, G.M.; Lipkin, M.E. Effect of Laser Settings and Irrigation Rates on Ureteral Temperature During Holmium Laser Lithotripsy, an In Vitro Model. *J. Endourol.* **2018**, *32*, 59–63. [CrossRef] [PubMed]
27. Aldoukhi, A.H.; Black, K.M.; Hall, T.L.; Ghani, K.R.; Maxwell, A.D.; MacConaghy, B.; Roberts, W.W. Defining thermally safe laser lithotripsy power and irrigation parameters: In vitro model. *J. Endourol.* **2020**, *34*, 76–81. [CrossRef] [PubMed]

Disclaimer/Publisher's Note: The statements, opinions and data contained in all publications are solely those of the individual author(s) and contributor(s) and not of MDPI and/or the editor(s). MDPI and/or the editor(s) disclaim responsibility for any injury to people or property resulting from any ideas, methods, instructions or products referred to in the content.

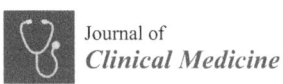

Article

Real Time Intrarenal Pressure Control during Flexible Ureterorrenscopy Using a Vascular PressureWire: Pilot Study

Alba Sierra [1,2,3], Mariela Corrales [2,3], Merkourios Kolvatzis [2,3,4], Steeve Doizi [2,3] and Olivier Traxer [2,3,*]

1. Urology Department, Hospital Clínic de Barcelona, Universitat de Barcelona, Villarroel 170, 08036 Barcelona, Spain
2. Sorbonne University GRC Urolithiasis No. 20 Tenon Hospital, F-75020 Paris, France
3. Department of Urology AP-HP, Tenon Hospital, Sorbonne University, F-75020 Paris, France
4. 2nd Department of Urology, Papageorgiou General Hospital, Aristotle University of Thessaloniki, 54124 Thessaloniki, Greece
* Correspondence: olivier.traxer@aphp.fr

Abstract: (1) Introduction: To evaluate the feasibility of measuring the intrapelvic pressure (IPP) during flexible ureterorenoscopy (f-URS) with a PressureWire and to optimize safety by assessing IPP during surgery. (2) Methods: Patients undergoing f-URS for different treatments were recruited. A PressureWire (0.014″, St. Jude Medical, Little Canada, MN, USA) was placed into the renal cavities to measure IPP. Gravity irrigation at 40 cmH$_2$O over the patient and a hand-assisted irrigation system were used. Pressures were monitored in real time and recorded for analysis. Fluid balance and postoperative urinary tract infection (UTI) were documented. (3) Results: Twenty patients undergoing f-URS were included with successful IPP monitoring. The median baseline IPP was 13.6 (6.8–47.6) cmH$_2$O. After the placement of the UAS, the median IPP was 17 (8–44.6) cmH$_2$O. With irrigation pressure set at 40 cmH$_2$O without forced irrigation, the median IPP was 34 (19–81.6) cmH$_2$O. Median IPP during laser lithotripsy, with and without the use of on-demand forced irrigation, was 61.2 (27.2–149.5) cmH$_2$O. The maximum pressure peaks recorded during forced irrigation ranged from 54.4 to 236.6 cmH$_2$O. After the surgery, 3 patients (15%) presented UTI; 2 of them had a positive preoperative urine culture, previously treated, and a positive fluid balance observed after the surgery. (4) Conclusion: Based on our experience, continuous monitoring of IPP with a wire is easy to reproduce, effective, and safe. In addition, it allows us to identify and avoid high IPPs, which may affect surgery-related complications.

Keywords: endourology; intrapelvic pressure; intrarenal pressure; ureteroscopy

1. Introduction

The development of fibre optic technology, digital ureteroscopes, and novel laser techniques have allowed the downsizing of flexible ureteroscopes, allowing not only treatment but also the diagnosis of many upper urinary tract conditions, such as kidney stones, ureteral strictures, and low-risk upper urothelial tumours [?,?]. Nevertheless, an adequate irrigation flow is required to achieve and maintain good visualization during these procedures [?].

With the downsizing of ureteroscopes, the working channel is typically reduced to 3.6 Fh. In endoscopic procedures, visibility is crucial, and it depends largely on the balance between the inflow, based on the irrigation pressure system and the working channel size, and the irrigation outflow, which depends on scope size and its relationship with the ureteral access sheath (UAS) [?]. The intrapelvic pressure (IPP) reached during f-URS is a result of irrigation inflow and outflow [?]. The physiological IPP ranges from 0 to 5 cmH$_2$O and the pyelo-venous backflow occurs at pressures of 40.8–47.6 cmH$_2$O [?,?]. During f-URS, when a disbalance occurs, high levels of IPP may be reached intraoperatively, causing pyelo-venous, and pyelo-lymphatic backflow or even rupture of the collecting system, possibly leading to peri-renal hematoma or urosepsis [?,?,?]. Prior in vivo studies have reported pressures as high as 436.9 cmH$_2$O during f-URS [?], massively exceeding the pressure of pyelovenous backflows.

Despite some clinical experiences [?] with the current endourology armamentarium, we are not able to measure real-time in vivo intrarenal pressure during endourological procedures. The aim of our study is to evaluate simultaneously the IPP values using a vascular PressureWire and avoid sudden pressure increases during different f-URS procedures.

2. Materials and Methods

2.1. Study Design

A prospective pilot study of consecutive patients undergoing f-URS for different treatments, including kidney stone disease, pyelo-ureteral junction syndrome (UPJ) and diagnosis/treatment for upper tract urothelial carcinoma (UTUC), was performed between March and April 2022

2.2. Method of IPP Measurement

The PressureWire (St. Jude Medical, Saint Paul, MN, USA) was used before by Doizi et al. for IPP monitoring [?]. This 0.014″ wire is approved and routinely used by cardiologists to assess fractional flow reserve in coronary arteries. The distal 3 cm of the wire, where the digital sensor is positioned to measure pressure, is made of soft platinum, which is floppy, radiopaque, hydrophilic and allows for positioning without renal trauma. In the following 28 cm, the wire is made of a polytetrafluoroethylene coating and is flexible and hydrophilic. Wirelessly, the pressure signal is transmitted to a console (QUANTIEN system) that displays the pressure (Figure ??). Pressure is recorded every second. The pressure is measured in mmHg and the available range is from -30 to 300 mmHg (-40.8 to 407.9 cmH$_2$O). Its accuracy is ± 1 mmHg plus $\pm 1\%$ ($\leq$50 mmHg) $\pm 3\%$ (>50 mmHg). Pressure values measured in mmHg were multiplied by 1.35951 to convert them in cmH$_2$O.

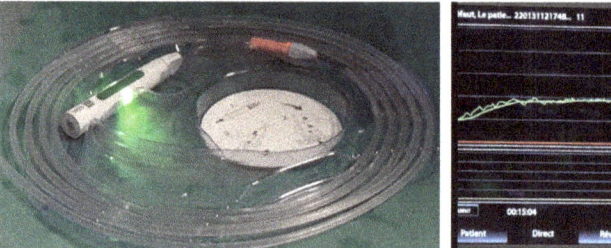
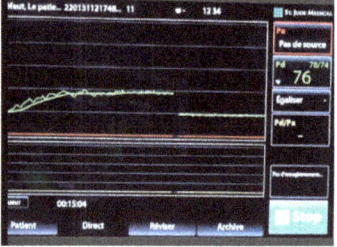

Figure 1. Wireless system. The PressureWire is activated by pressing a button (green light) and automatically connected wirelessly to a console (QUANTIEN system). The zeroing must be completed before the PressureWire placement, outside the patient. Once it is connected, it starts to simultaneously transmit the pressure signal to the screen.

2.3. Procedures

Perioperative antibiotic prophylaxis was administrated following the local protocol. All procedures were performed under general anaesthesia. Each procedure began with a cystoscopy and the placement of a hydrophilic guidewire in the renal pelvis under fluoroscopic guidance. A dual lumen ureteral catheter (Cook Medical, Bloomington, IN, USA) was then inserted and the PressureWire was placed in the renal pelvis for IPP measurements (Figure ??). Once the dual lumen catheter was removed, the f-URS was either passed directly over the hydrophilic guidewire or, when indicated, through a UAS inserted over the hydrophilic guidewire (Retrace 10/12 or 12/14, 35 cm, Coloplast, Humlebaek, Denmark). In some cases, PressureWire was placed into the UAS (Figure ??). Retrograde intrarenal surgery (RIRS) was performed using a flexible digital re-usable ureteroscope, the Flex—Xc (Karl Storz, Tuttlingen, Germany), with a constant 0.9% saline irrigation pressure (40 cmH$_2$O) at ambient temperature and a manual pump (Traxerflow Dual Port, Rocamed, Monaco), allowing on-demand forced irrigation when a better view was required. All of the interventions performed by an experienced endourologist (OT). The assistant controlled the pressure during the entire surgery, ensuring good vision and trying not to exceed values above 60 cmH$_2$O (Figure **??**). When laser treatment was needed, a thulium fibre laser (SOLTIVE Premium, Olympus, Tokio, Japan or FIBERDUST, Quanta System, Samarate, Italy) was used. At the end of each surgery, we inserted a ureteral stent (Double J) for 7–10 days. Patients were followed in the postoperative period to identify any possible complications.

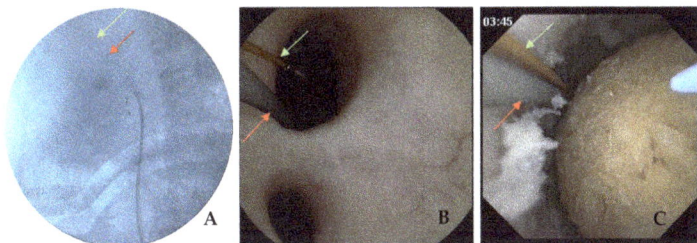

Figure 2. Pressure wire placement intro renal pelvis: (**A**) fluoroscopic image of PressureWire (green) and safety wire (red) in the renal pelvis. (**B**) Endoscopic vision of the renal pelvis with a PressureWire (green) and safety wire (red) going inside the upper calyx. (**C**) Endoscopic vision before starting lithotripsy of a dihydrate calcium oxalate stone with a safety wire (red), PressureWire (green) and fibre laser in the renal pelvis.

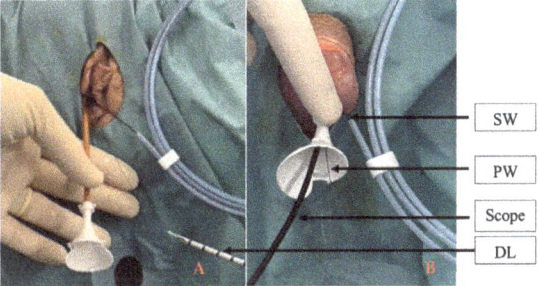

Figure 3. (**A**) Placement of PressureWire after the use of a dual lumen ureteral access catheter (Cook Medical, Germany). (**B**) PressureWire was placed through the UAS (Retrace 10/12, 35 cm, Coloplast, Denmark) with a digital reusable flexible ureterorenoscope (Flex-XC, 8.5Fh, Storz, Germany) inside. SW, safety wire. PW, PressureWire. DL, dual lumen.

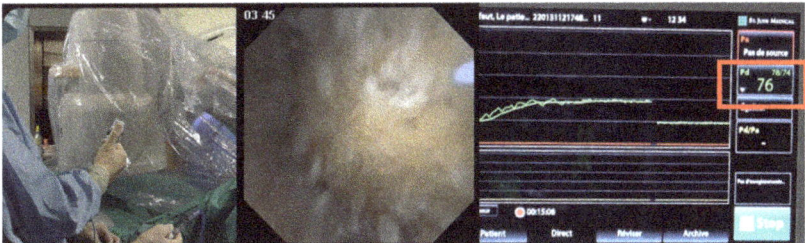

Figure 4. Pressure is simultaneously transmitted to the screen during endoscopic procedure. The pressure is measured in mmHg and the available range is from −30 to 300 mmHg. In this figure, during manual assisted irrigation (Traxerflow Dual Port, Rocamed, Monaco), we achieve IPP at 76 mmHg.

2.4. Data Collection

- Baseline IPP: recorded with only the PressureWire in place, prior to f-URS insertion and irrigation flow.
- UAS IPP: Recorded when placing the UAS
- Scope IPP: Recorded during the introduction of the flexible ureteroscope into the renal cavities and irrigation pressure set at 40 cmH2O without any forced irrigation.
- Therapeutic period IPP: Once reaching a plateau for 30 s. In real time, the assistant responsible for forced irrigation was aware of IPP measurements.

In case of stone disease, patients underwent non-contrast-enhanced CT for stone volume, which was obtained with the formula of an ellipsoid ($4/3 \times \pi \times$ radius length $\times$ radius width $\times$ radius depth). Median IPP values, peak pressures, and pressure patterns with and without the scope in the renal cavity were examined, as well as the influence of on-demand irrigation during the surgical procedure. The fluid balance (FB) was the difference between the saline irrigation volume used during the surgery and the volume in the vacuum at the end of the surgery. During the hospitalisation, postoperative complications were recorded. For statistical analysis, categorical variables were measured as percentages and numerical variables were expressed as medians (interquartile range (IQR)).

3. Results

Of the 20 patients included in this study, 55% (n = 11) were male and 45 (n = 9) female. The median age was 51 (19–79) years old. Placement of the PressureWire succeeded in all cases and IPP measurements were obtained in all cases (Table ??).

Two patients with UTUC, one for surveillance and the other one for endoscopic treatment, had baseline pressures of 15 cmH_2O in both cases. Therapeutic IPP was 57 cmH_2O. However, the maximum peak pressure recorder was 114.2 cmH_2O.

One patient with pyelo-ureteral junction syndrome demonstrated a pressure two times higher than the baseline pressure after the administration of furosemide iv (1 mg).

f-URS was performed for stone lithotripsy in 85% of cases (n = 17). Four of them were pre-stented. The median stone burden was 864 (50–9000) mm^3. Overall, 52% (n = 9) were calcium oxalate stones. The median baseline IPP was 13.6 (6.8–47.6) cmH_2O. UAS was used in 14 patients (70%), mostly 10/12 Fr, according to the surgeon's choice. After UAS placement, the median UAS IPP was 17 (8–44.6) cmH_2O. During f-URS, with the endoscope in the renal cavity and irrigation pressure set at 40 cmH_2O without any forced irrigation, the median IPP was 37.4 (19–81.6) cmH_2O when UAS was used and 35.2 (21.8–64) cmH_2O without UAS. We controlled the pressure simultaneously during all of the surgeries. When forced irrigation was used, immediate IPP changes were observed, according to the way in which the assistant used the irrigation system. The median IPP during therapeutic period with the use of on-demand forced irrigation was 61.2 (27.2–149.5) cmH_2O. The maximum pressure peaks recorded during this period ranged from 54.4 to 238 cmH_2O.

The median surgery time was 149.5 (60–256) min. Positive preoperative urine culture was detected in 25% (n = 5) patients, all of them with renal stones (Table ??). According to the antibiogram, antibiotherapy was started 3 days before the surgery in all cases. Overall, 15% (n = 3) of patients were diagnosed with a UTI after the procedure. The complication rate was low and mostly Clavien–Dindo grade I and II. There were no complications related to PressureWire placement.

Table 1. Patient characteristics and intrapelvic pressures during flexible ureteroscopy.

Patient	Treatment	Stone Burden (mm³)	Stone Type	Pre-Stented	Fibre Size (μm)	UAS Size (Fr)	IPP (cmH$_2$O)			Therapeutic Period	Maximum Pressure Peak
							Baseline	UAS	Scope		
1	Lithotripsy	9000	Cystine	Yes	200	10/12	47.6	44.6	40.8	54.4	163
2	Lithotripsy	7500	Infective	No	200	10/12	20.4	21.3	68	68	197
3	Lithotripsy	3190	Infective	No	200	10/12	16.3	20.4	27.2	68	176.7
4	Lithotripsy	864	Carbapatite	No	200	10/12	16.3	18.2	19	27.2	54.4
5			Pyeloureteral junction syndrome		No		13.6			30 (furosemide)	
6	Lithotripsy	3000	Cystine	Yes	272	10/12	13.6	15	81.6	136	238
7			Upper tract urinary tumour (diagnosis)		No		15	No	30	No	15
8	Lithotripsy	6000	OCD	Yes	200	10/12	20.4	27.2	61.2	149.5	236.6
9			Upper tract urinary tumour (treatment)		272	No	15	No	15	No	34
10	Lithotripsy	864	OCM	No	200	12/14	21.8	24.5	51.7	110.1	171.3
11	Lithotripsy	4000	OCD	No	200	10/12	13.6	13.6	31.3	54.4	99.2
12	Lithotripsy	5410	OCD	No	150	10/12	12.2	16.3	47.6	117	156.3
13	Lithotripsy	740	Mixed	No	200	10/12	12.2	13.6	20.4	70.7	122.4
14	Lithotripsy	270	OCD	No	200	No	13.6	No	64	93.8	206.4
15	Lithotripsy	260	OCM	No	150	10/12	13.6	13.6	45	54.4	163.1
16	Lithotripsy	50	OCM		No		6.8	No	6.8	No	26.4
17	Lithotripsy	550	Brushite	Yes	150	12/14	13.6	13.6	27.2	34	84.3
18	Lithotripsy	431	OCM	No	200	No	9.5	No	21.8	61.2	102
19	Lithotripsy	4000	OCD	No	150	10/12	9.5	8.1	34	61.2	119.6
20	Lithotripsy	658	OCD	Yes	150	10/12	15.0	17.6	27.2	34	69.3

OCD: oxalate calcium dehydrate. OCM: oxalate calcium monohydrate.

Table 2. Relationship between peak pressure, fluid absorption and postoperative complications.

Patient	Preoperative Urine Culture	Surgery Time (min)	Peak Pressure (cmH$_2$O)	Fluid Balance (mL)	Postoperative Infection	Clavien–Dindo (<1 month)
1	Sterile	164	163	0	No	I
2	S. agalactia (Cefotaxime)	210	197	+300	Fever (4 days)	II
3	Sterile	145	176.7	+600	No	I
4	E. coli (Amoxicillin)	160	54.4	0	No	I
5	Sterile	120	30	0	No	I
6	Sterile	167	238	−100	No	O I
7	Sterile	102	15	−500	No	I
8	P. aeruginosa (Meropenem)	256	236.6	+650	No	I
9	Sterile	208	34	0	No	I
10	Sterile	147	171.3	−400	Outpatient	I
11	Sterile	185	99.2	−500	No	I
12	Sterile	117	156.3	+400	No	I
13	Sterile	135	122.4	0	Outpatient	I
14	Sterile	105	206.4	0	No	I
15	Sterile	199	163.1	+600	Fever (7 days)	II
16	Sterile	113	26.4	−200	Outpatient	I
17	S. aureus (Bactrim)	178	84.3	0	Fever (2 days)	II
18	Sterile	121	102	+500	Outpatient	I
19	P. aeruginosa (Tienam)	152	119.6	0	No	I
20	Sterile	60	69.3	0	No	I

4. Discussion

Pyelovenous backflow, which occurs at pressures of 40.8–47.6 cmH$_2$O, is an event that most urologists try to avoid [?,?]. That is why an IPP around 40 cmH$_2$O is recognised as an aspirational threshold and should be the goal during endourological procedures [?]. In our pilot study, although IPP was rigorously controlled, maintaining IPP around 40 cmH$_2$O was not feasible to maintain good visualization. We target pressures as low as possible, achieving 61.2 cmH$_2$O median IPP. In a recent systematic review, IPP at 40 cmH$_2$O was also exceeded during ureterorenoscopic procedures, specially without UAS [?]. Additionally, if we consider high-power laser lithotripsy, moderate irrigation is needed for the laser to be safe, because if irrigation rates decrease, we can produce a significant temperature increase, potentially resulting in urothelial tissue injuries [?]. Understanding this fact is crucial when interpreting findings, since improving drainage may be preferable compared to decreasing irrigation pressure/flow.

Unlike prior in vivo human studies where a ureteral catheter or a nephrostomy tube were used [?,?], we placed a 0.014″ PressureWire in renal cavities. This IPP method measurement was described previously by Doizi et al. [?]. This system offers several advantages: it can be used for endoscopic procedures with all scope brands, and as the wire is placed into renal cavities, we can control IPP throughout the the procedure, because in addition to working along the ureter to treat, e.g.., a ureteral stone, which is important, it can work up to the pyeloureteral junction [?,?]. However, its small size prevents us from using it as a safety wire, needing us to place both the PressureWire and a safety wire.

Regardless of the IPP measurement method, with gravity irrigation at 40 cmH$_2$O, similar baseline IPPs were also reported in the literature, ranging from 23.8 to 57 cmH$_2$O without UAS and 13.14 to 33.99 cmH$_2$O with a 10/12 UAS [?]. In addition, the scope IPP without UAS was two to three times higher than baseline IPP, which demonstrates once again that higher IPP is achieved without UAS [?]. Concerning therapeutic IPP, no comparison can be performed with previous studies, since many parameters differ: f-URS model, gravity and forced irrigation, pre-stenting and use or not of UAS and its size.

Prior in vivo human studies have reported peak pressures above 400 cmH$_2$O [? ? ?]. In our cohort, by means of simultaneous IPP control, we halved these values for a short period of time. By means of simultaneous IPP control, we can quicky react to decreased IPP, avoiding pathological kidney changes reported in the literature [?]. In this line, in the immediate follow-up, no urinary extravasation was identified. However, fluid absorption was noted in four patients. Fluid absorption during f-URS usually remains low, mainly due to the smaller instrument calibre and the small irrigation channel. Nevertheless, increasing the flow to maintain optimal visibility necessitates the use of high-pressure irrigation, thus increasing the risk of fluid extravasation. IPP is not the only parameter to consider during fluid absorption; urothelial damage and surgery length are also important. Cybulski et al. reported that there is approximately 1 mL of irrigation fluid absorbed per minute of URS time at 271.9 cmH$_2$O [?].

Additionally, the procedure time is independently correlated with increased postoperative fever and SIRS rates [?]. There is probably a correlation between IPP and infectious complications such as UTI and sepsis during endourological procedures, as well as other factors such as patient age, stone size and type, and length of the surgery [? ?]. For instance, 15% of the patients in our series presented with postoperative UTI despite therapeutic IPP at 40 cmH$_2$O, meaning that other factors may contribute to the development of infectious complications.

We are convinced that the next step to improve safety during intrarenal procedures will be IPP monitoring. In this line, the recently developed LithoVueTM Elite System (BostonScientific, Boston, MA, USA) might contribute to safety and will provide us with more information about intrarenal pressure during endourologic procedures. However, for now, this new device needs to be evaluated, since the post-market study recently started in July 2022. Moreover, as the pressure sensor is located on the scope's tip, to measure IPP we will need the scope to be placed inside the kidney, while with the PressureWire we can control IPP throughout the procedure. In future research, it will be interesting to compare both methods of pressure monitoring.

5. Conclusions

In our experience, the use of the PressureWire for IPP measurement during therapeutic and diagnosis f-URS is simple, safe, reproducible, and independent of the f-URS procedure. Continuously monitoring the IPP in real time allows us to identify and avoid high IPPs, which may lead to surgery-related complications.

Author Contributions: Conceptualization, O.T. and S.D.; methodology, O.T.; formal analysis, M.C.; investigation, A.S. and M.K.; data curation, M.K.; writing—original draft preparation, A.S.; writing—review and editing, M.C.; supervision, O.T. All authors have read and agreed to the published version of the manuscript.

Funding: This research received no external funding.

Institutional Review Board Statement: Ethical review and approval were waived for this study, due to prior published paper using same PressureWire in humans.

Informed Consent Statement: Informed consent was obtained from all subjects involved in the study.

Data Availability Statement: Data is unavailable due to privacy.

Conflicts of Interest: Alba Sierra, Mariela Corrales and Merkourios Kolvatzis have nothing to disclose. Olivier Traxer is a consultant for Boston Scientific, Coloplast, EMS, IPG, Quanta and Rocamed, but has no specific conflicts relevant to this work.

References

1. Proietti, S.; Knoll, T.; Giusti, G. Contemporary ureteroscopic management of renal stones. *Int. J. Surg.* **2016**, *36*, 681–687. [CrossRef] [PubMed]
2. Türk, C.; Petřík, A.; Sarica, K.; Seitz, C.; Skolarikos, A.; Straub, M.; Knoll, T. EAU Guidelines on Interventional Treatment for Urolithiasis. *Eur. Urol.* **2016**, *69*, 475–482. [CrossRef] [PubMed]
3. Schwalb, D.M.; Eshghi, M.; Ian, M.D.; Franco, I. Morphological and Physiological Changes in the Urinary Tract Associated with Ureteral Dilation and Ureteropyeloscopy: An Experimental Study. *J. Urol.* **1993**, *149*, 1576–1585. [CrossRef] [PubMed]
4. Sener, T.E.; Cloutier, J.; Villa, L.; Marson, F.; Butticè, S.; Doizi, S.; Traxer, O. Can We Provide Low Intrarenal Pressures with Good Irrigation Flow by Decreasing the Size of Ureteral Access Sheaths? *J. Endourol.* **2016**, *30*, 49–55, Erratum in *J. Endourol.* **2017**, *31*, 110. [CrossRef] [PubMed]
5. Hinman, F.; Redewill, F.H. Pyelovenous back flow. *JAMA* **1926**, *87*, 1287–1293. [CrossRef]
6. Kiil, F. Pressure recordings in the upper urinary tract. *Scand. J. Clin. Lab. Investig.* **1953**, *5*, 383–384. [CrossRef] [PubMed]
7. Xu, L.; Li, G. Life-threatening subcapsular renal hematoma after flexible ureteroscopic laser lithotripsy: Treatment with superselective renal arterial embolization. *Urolithiasis* **2013**, *41*, 449–451. [CrossRef] [PubMed]
8. Stenberg, A.; Bohman, S.-O.; Morsing, P.; Müller-Suur, C.; Olsen, L.; Persson, A.E.G. Back-leak of pelvic urine to the bloodstream. *Acta Physiol. Scand.* **1988**, *134*, 223–234. [CrossRef] [PubMed]
9. Doizi, S.; Letendre, J.; Cloutier, J.; Ploumidis, A.; Traxer, O. Continuous monitoring of intrapelvic pressure during flexible ureteroscopy using a sensor wire: A pilot study. *World J. Urol.* **2021**, *39*, 555–561. [CrossRef] [PubMed]
10. Croghan, S.M.; Skolarikos, A.; Jack, G.S.; Manecksha, R.P.; Walsh, M.T.; O'Brien, F.J.; Davis, N.F. Upper urinary tract pressures in endourology: A systematic review of range, variables and implications. *BJU Int.* **2022**; *ahead of print*. [CrossRef]
11. Chiron, P.; Mandé, S.; Doizi, S.; De Coninck, V.; Keller, E.X.; Berthe, L.; Traxer, O. MP17-04 evaluation of heat generation in an in vitro kidney model: Does the superpulsed thulium fiber laser pose a risk? *J. Urol.* **2019**, *201* (Suppl. 4), e256. [CrossRef]
12. Auge, B.K.; Pietrow, P.K.; Preminger, G.M. 1890: The Ureteral Access Sheath Provides Protection Against Elevated Intra-Renal Pressures Generated During Routine Flexible Ureteroscopic Stone Manipulation. *J. Urol.* **2004**, *171*, 499. [CrossRef]
13. Jung, H.; Osther, P.J. Intraluminal pressure profiles during flexible ureterorenoscopy. *SpringerPlus* **2015**, *4*, 373. [CrossRef] [PubMed]
14. Tokas, T.; Herrmann, T.R.W.; Skolarikos, A.; Nagele, U. Pressure matters: Intrarenal pressures during normal and pathological conditions, and impact of increased values to renal physiology. *World J. Urol.* **2019**, *37*, 125–131. [CrossRef] [PubMed]
15. Cybulski, P.; Honey, R.J.D.; Pace, K. Fluid Absorption during Ureterorenoscopy. *J. Endourol.* **2004**, *18*, 739–742. [CrossRef] [PubMed]
16. Zhong, W.; Leto, G.; Wang, L.; Zeng, G. Systemic Inflammatory Response Syndrome After Flexible Ureteroscopic Lithotripsy: A Study of Risk Factors. *J. Endourol.* **2015**, *29*, 25–28. [CrossRef] [PubMed]
17. Lane, J.; Whitehurst, L.; Hameed, B.Z.; Tokas, T.; Somani, B.K. Correlation of Operative Time with Outcomes of Ureteroscopy and Stone Treatment: A Systematic Review of Literature. *Curr. Urol. Rep.* **2020**, *21*, 17. [CrossRef] [PubMed]

Disclaimer/Publisher's Note: The statements, opinions and data contained in all publications are solely those of the individual author(s) and contributor(s) and not of MDPI and/or the editor(s). MDPI and/or the editor(s) disclaim responsibility for any injury to people or property resulting from any ideas, methods, instructions or products referred to in the content.

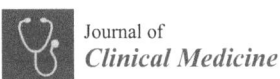

Article

Factors Affecting the Usage of Wearable Device Technology for Healthcare among Indian Adults: A Cross-Sectional Study

Vathsala Patil [1], Deepak Kumar Singhal [2,*], Nithesh Naik [3,4,5,*], B. M. Zeeshan Hameed [4,5,6], Milap J. Shah [4,7], Sufyan Ibrahim [4,8], Komal Smriti [1], Gaurav Chatterjee [9], Ameya Kale [10], Anshika Sharma [11], Rahul Paul [4,12,13], Piotr Chłosta [14] and Bhaskar K. Somani [15]

1. Department of Oral Medicine and Radiology, Manipal College of Dental Sciences, Manipal, Manipal Academy of Higher Education, Manipal 576104, Karnataka, India
2. Department of Public Health Dentistry, Manipal College of Dental Sciences, Manipal, Manipal Academy of Higher Education, Manipal 576104, Karnataka, India
3. Department of Mechanical and Industrial Engineering, Manipal Institute of Technology, Manipal Academy of Higher Education, Manipal 576104, Karnataka, India
4. iTRUE (International Training and Research in Uro-Oncology and Endourology) Group, Manipal 576104, Karnataka, India
5. Curiouz TechLab Private Limited, BIRAC-BioNEST, Government of Karnataka Bioincubator, Manipal 576104, Karnataka, India
6. Department of Urology, Father Muller Medical College, Mangalore 575001, Karnataka, India
7. Robotics and Urooncology, Max Hospital and Max Institute of Cancer Care, New Delhi 110024, India
8. Department of Neurosurgery, Mayo Clinic, Rochester, MN 55902, USA
9. Department of Electrical and Electronics Engineering, Manipal Institute of Technology, Manipal Academy of Higher Education, Manipal 576104, Karnataka, India
10. Kasturba Medical College, Manipal, Manipal Academy of Higher Education, Manipal 576104, Karnataka, India
11. Department of Psychology, Amity University, Noida 201313, Uttar Pradesh, India
12. Department of Radiation Oncology, Massachusetts General Hospital, Harvard Medical School, Boston, MA 02114, USA
13. Center for Biologics Evaluation and Research (CBER), U.S. Food and Drug Administration, Silver Spring, MD 20993, USA
14. Department of Urology, Jagiellonian University in Krakow, 31-007 Kraków, Poland
15. Department of Urology, University Hospital Southampton NHS Trust, Southampton SO16 6YD, UK
* Correspondence: dk.singhal@manipal.edu (D.K.S.); nithesh.naik@manipal.edu (N.N.); Tel.: +91-8310874339 (N.N.)

Abstract: Background: Wearable device technology has recently been involved in the healthcare industry substantially. India is the world's third largest market for wearable devices and is projected to expand at a compound annual growth rate of ~26.33%. However, there is a paucity of literature analyzing the factors determining the acceptance of wearable healthcare device technology among low-middle-income countries. Methods: This cross-sectional, web-based survey aims to analyze the perceptions affecting the adoption and usage of wearable devices among the Indian population aged 16 years and above. Results: A total of 495 responses were obtained. In all, 50.3% were aged between 25–50 years and 51.3% belonged to the lower-income group. While 62.2% of the participants reported using wearable devices for managing their health, 29.3% were using them daily. technology and task fitness (TTF) showed a significant positive correlation with connectivity ($r = 0.716$), health care ($r = 0.780$), communication ($r = 0.637$), infotainment ($r = 0.598$), perceived usefulness (PU) ($r = 0.792$), and perceived ease of use (PEOU) ($r = 0.800$). Behavioral intention (BI) to use wearable devices positively correlated with PEOU ($r = 0.644$) and PU ($r = 0.711$). All factors affecting the use of wearable devices studied had higher mean scores among participants who were already using wearable devices. Male respondents had significantly higher mean scores for BI ($p = 0.034$) and PEOU ($p = 0.009$). Respondents older than 25 years of age had higher mean scores for BI ($p = 0.027$) and Infotainment ($p = 0.032$). Conclusions: This study found a significant correlation with the adoption and acceptance of wearable devices for healthcare management in the Indian context.

Citation: Patil, V.; Singhal, D.K.; Naik, N.; Hameed, B.M.Z.; Shah, M.J.; Ibrahim, S.; Smriti, K.; Chatterjee, G.; Kale, A.; Sharma, A.; et al. Factors Affecting the Usage of Wearable Device Technology for Healthcare among Indian Adults: A Cross-Sectional Study. *J. Clin. Med.* **2022**, *11*, 7019. https://doi.org/10.3390/jcm11237019

Academic Editor: Enrico Checcucci

Received: 21 October 2022
Accepted: 24 November 2022
Published: 28 November 2022

Publisher's Note: MDPI stays neutral with regard to jurisdictional claims in published maps and institutional affiliations.

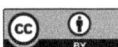

Copyright: © 2022 by the authors. Licensee MDPI, Basel, Switzerland. This article is an open access article distributed under the terms and conditions of the Creative Commons Attribution (CC BY) license (https://creativecommons.org/licenses/by/4.0/).

Keywords: wearable healthcare devices; fitness devices; wearable technology; infotainment; mobile health

1. Introduction

Wearable devices are instruments that can be worn on the body, typically on or near the skin, and are equipped with sensors capable of detecting various physiological variables. Wearable technology includes devices that can be placed on the limbs, torso, or head such as watches, bracelets, phones, glasses, head-mounted displays, hearing aids, suits, belts, shoes, and patches that can measure various physiological parameters, which include heart rate, rhythm, blood pressure, oxygen saturation, skin temperature, steps traveled, calorie expenditure estimates, blood glucose levels, and UV radiation exposure [1]. This data can be used for physiological-related research studies, detection of aberrant parameters for clinical diagnosis or prognosis to provide biological feedback to the user thereby aiding in monitoring, and even as an educational tool for promoting health and physical fitness. One of the earliest examples of wearable technology, as it pertains to the field of medicine, are portable hearing aids invented in the 19th century [2]. Norman Holter's discovery of the first wireless electrocardiogram in 1962 ushered in the era of modern medical wearable gadgets [3,4]. The internet enables health-directed wearable devices to stay connected while continuously measuring and recording data. This system is now referred to as "Connected Health" [5].

Newer studies have aimed at early identification and prediction of inflammatory disease, cancer diagnosis, measuring blood alcohol levels, etc. through smartphone screens. Combining deep neural network-machine learning technology with biological age estimation has further enhanced its feasibility and usage [6–10]. In recent years, the world has seen a wave of adoption of wearable devices even among the middle to high-income socio-economic demographics. A recent systematic review and meta-analysis of multiple randomized controlled trials of consumer wearable activity trackers (CWAT) found that they can improve physical activity in sedentary older adults who are overweight/obese or with chronic respiratory diseases and reduce the systolic blood pressure, waist circumference and low-density cholesterol in individuals with type 2 diabetes mellitus and cardiovascular diseases [11]. Wearable devices such as smartwatches have been seen to benefit psychological wellness in individuals with cognitive disorders [12].

India is now the world's third-largest market for wearable devices. Several studies have found that an increasing number of individuals are purchasing wearable devices to promote fitness and manage their health [13,14]. A recent study determined that consumers in India are motivated by health and autonomy, health self-efficacy, and technological innovativeness to adopt wearable healthcare devices [15,16]. The COVID-19 pandemic encouraged a rapid, massive expansion of remote health management and firmly established telehealth as an accessible, validated model of healthcare. The data on the pandemic's effect on actual wearable device use in healthcare settings is limited. Studies examining the perception of wearable device technology among adults in India are limited in the literature. Hence, the present study aimed to analyze the perception of Indian Professionals about wearable device technology in terms of its usage in personal health management.

2. Materials and Methods

2.1. Data Collection and Ethical Considerations

A cross-sectional study was carried out from January 2022 to May 2022 using an online questionnaire, using an anonymized Google form platform, enquiring about participants' use of wearable devices for healthcare, socio-demographic factors, and factors affecting the use of wearable devices for healthcare. The technology acceptance model (TAM) and technology and task fitness (TTF) models of technology adoption were used for the survey. Data acquisition and analysis were performed after the approval by the Institutional Ethical committee (ethical approval number FMIEC- 94/2021). Informed consent was obtained from all the participants before the study and the data was analyzed by an independent third party.

The questionnaire gathered information regarding demographics, behavioral intention (BI), perceived usefulness (PU), perceived ease of use (PEOU), subjective feelings about technology, task fitness, connectivity, communication, healthcare, infotainment, fashionability, wearability, and subjective norms. The questionnaire (available as Supplementary Materials) was divided into 11 sections, with 3 items each directed at identifying the subject's feelings concerning wearable devices according to factors described in the TAM model and factors derived from the TTF models, and was distributed to the participants. The response was documented based on a 5-point answer choice based on the Likert scale as follows: (1)—Strongly Disagree/Very Rarely, (2)—Disagree/Rarely, (3)—Undecided/Occasionally, (4)—Agree/Often, and (5)—Strongly Agree/Very Often.

2.2. Survey and Participant Characteristics

Respondents consisted majorly of individuals involved in medical science (undergraduate students, postgraduates, consultant physicians) and the engineering field. The questionnaire was surveyed using the Google Forms platform, which focused on the perception and stated usage of wearable devices by the participants. The inclusion criteria for the study included adults >16 years, able to navigate through the online survey platforms, and comfortable with the interpretation of the English language. An information sheet along with informed consent was displayed and documented respectively at the start of the survey. Participation in this survey was voluntary with no incentives provided to the respondents. Survey data collected via Google Forms was stored on the Google Spreadsheet platform on Google Drive, access to which was limited only to members of the research group.

2.3. Data Analysis

The responses to the survey were analyzed using the SmartPLS software version 3.0.M3, with PLS path modeling. Descriptive variables of gender, age, qualification, income, and reports of usage of wearable devices for personal healthcare were expressed as categorical variables. Age data were grouped according to less than 18 years old, 18 to 25 years old, 25 to 50 years old, and older than 50 years. Qualification data were grouped according to (1) "10 + 2 schooling", (2) "graduate", (3) "post-graduate", and (4) "diploma" categories. Income data were grouped from a personal annual income of (1) less than 50,000 Rs to 500,000 Rs. (Lower), (2) 500,000 to 2,500,000 Rs. (Middle), (3) 2,500,000 to 5,000,000 Rs. (Upper Middle) and (4) greater than 5,000,000 Rs. (Elite). Wearable device use-frequency data was grouped into (1) once a year, (2) more than once a year, (3) once in a month, (4) once or twice in 3 months, (5) once or twice in a week, and (6) daily. Wearable device usage for healthcare was assessed using a binary "yes" or "no" response. Usage frequency data were grouped according to (1) daily, (2) once or twice in a week, (3) once in a month, (4) once or twice in 3 months, (5) more than once a year, and (6) once a year.

Correlation between technology-task fitness and connectivity, communication, healthcare, infotainment, perceived usefulness, and perceived ease of use was tested by calculation of the Pearson correlation coefficient with a 2-tailed significance level set at 5% (alpha < 0.05). Pearson correlation coefficient was calculated with a 2-tailed significance level set at 5% (alpha < 0.05) between behavioral intention and fashionability, s, Subjective norms, perceived usefulness, and perceived ease of use. An independent sample t-test was performed to compare mean scores of all factors in respondents who reported using wearable devices for healthcare versus those who reported not using them, to compare male versus female respondents, and between the less than 25 years age group and more than 25 years age group ($p < 0.05$). Figure 1 shows the proposed research model with the various factors considered to evaluate the influence of the usage or barriers of wearable device technology for healthcare.

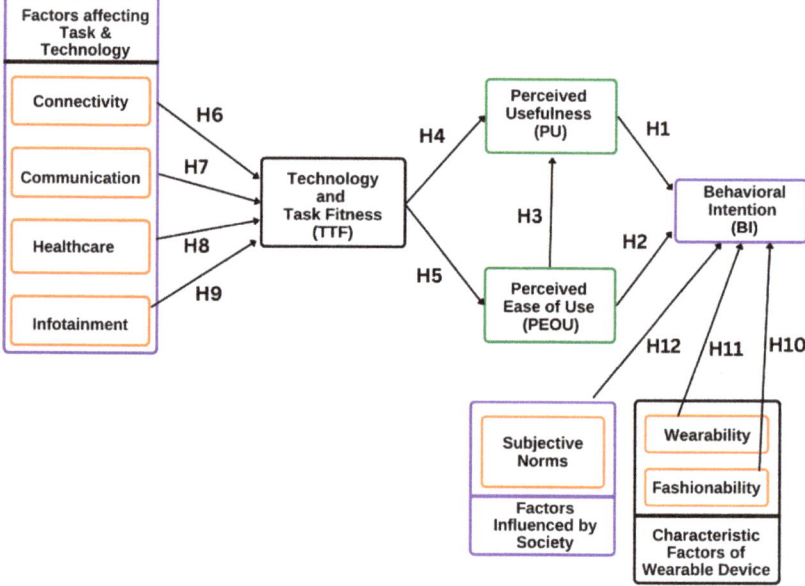

Figure 1. Proposed research model.

3. Results

A total of 495 responses were obtained from the Google form questionnaire. General data for the participants are as follows: 65.5% of respondents were male and 34.5% were females; 50.3% were between 25–50 years of age; 51.3% reported being in the lower-income group (annual income less than Rs. 50,000 to Rs. 500,000); 62.2% of participants reported already using wearable devices for managing their health; 29.3% reported using wearable devices daily. Table 1 shows the demographic characteristics of the participants considered in the present study.

Table 1. Demographic characteristics of study participants.

Variables		Number of Participants	Percentage (%)
Gender	Male	324	65.5
	Female	171	34.5
Age (in Years)	Less than 18	22	4.4
	18–25	186	37.6
	25–50	249	50.3
	More than 50	38	7.7
Income	Lower (Less than 50,000–500,000)	254	51.3
	Middle (500,000–2,500,000)	172	34.7
	Upper Middle (2,500,000–5,000,000)	44	8.9
	Elite (Greater than 5,000,000)	25	5.1
Are you currently using wearable devices for your healthcare?	No	187	37.8
	Yes	308	62.2
How frequently do you use wearable healthcare devices?	Once a year	145	29.3
	More than once a year	33	6.7
	Once a month	62	12.5
	Once or twice in 3 months	39	7.9
	Once or twice a week	71	14.3
	Daily	145	29.3

It was found that TTF moderately positively correlated with communication ($r = 0.637$) and infotainment ($r = 0.598$) and highly positively correlated with connectivity ($r = 0.716$) and health care ($r = 0.780$). Perceived usefulness ($r = 0.792$) and perceived ease of use ($r = 0.800$) were also found to be strongly correlated. Behavioral intention to use wearable devices was positively correlated to factors such as perceived usefulness, perceived ease of use, fashionability, wearability, and subjective norms. However, it was mildly correlated with fashionability ($r = 0.472$), moderately correlated with wearability ($r = 0.642$), subjective norms ($r = 0.594$), and perceived ease of use ($r = 0.644$), and highly correlated with perceived usefulness ($r = 0.711$). Table 2 shows the correlation values of the respective factors affecting technology and task fitness and behavioral intention in using wearable devices.

Table 2. Factors affecting technology and task fitness (TTF) and Behavioral Intention to use Wearable Devices [N = 495].

Variable	Pearson Correlation	Sig. (2-Tailed)
Technology and Task Fitness		
Connectivity	0.716 **	<0.001
Communication	0.637 **	<0.001
Health Care	0.780 **	<0.001
Infotainment	0.598 **	<0.001
Perceived Usefulness	0.792 **	<0.001
Perceived Ease of Use	0.800 **	<0.001
Behavioral Intention		
Fashionability	472 **	<0.001
Wearability	0.642 **	<0.001
Subjective Norms	0.594 **	<0.001
Perceived Usefulness	0.711 **	<0.001
Perceived Ease of Use	0.644 **	<0.001

** Correlation is significant at the 0.01 level (2-tailed).

Table 3 shows that all factors have significantly higher mean scores among those participants who are already using wearable devices as compared to non-users ($p < 0.001$). There is no significant difference in mean scores of all the variables among the males and females except for behavioral intention to use wearable devices and perceived ease of use of devices. Males have significantly higher mean scores for behavioral intention ($p = 0.034$) and perceived ease of use ($p = 0.009$). There is no significant difference in mean scores of any of the variables among the two different age groups except for behavioral intention to use wearable devices and infotainment. The participants who are more than 25 years old have significantly higher mean scores for behavioral intention ($p = 0.027$) and infotainment ($p = 0.032$).

Table 3. Mean scores of different factors affecting the use of wearable devices across already usage of wearable devices, gender, and age.

Variables	Already Using Wearable Devices for Healthcare		p-Value	Gender		p-Value	Age		p-Value
	Yes (N = 308)	No (N = 187)		Male (N = 324)	Female (N = 171)		Less than 25 Years (N = 207)	More than 25 Years (N = 287)	
	Mean (SD)	Mean (SD)		Mean (SD)	Mean (SD)		Mean (SD)	Mean (SD)	
Behavioral Intention	12.47 (2.4)	10.88 (3.1)	<0.001 *	12.06 (2.6)	11.50 (3.1)	0.034 *	11.54 (2.6)	12.11 (2.9)	0.027 *
Perceived Usefulness	13.09 (2.3)	10.43 (3.4)	<0.001 *	12.20 (2.9)	11.86 (3.4)	0.24	11.83 (2.9)	12.26 (3.1)	0.122
Perceived Ease of Use	13.36 (2.2)	11.17 (3.7)	<0.001 *	12.79 (2.8)	12.04 (3.4)	0.009 *	12.51 (3.0)	12.54 (3.0)	0.910

Table 3. Cont.

Variables	Already Using Wearable Devices for Healthcare		p-Value	Gender		p-Value	Age		p-Value
	Yes (N = 308)	No (N = 187)		Male (N = 324)	Female (N = 171)		Less Than 25 Years (N = 207)	More Than 25 Years (N = 287)	
	Mean (SD)	Mean (SD)		Mean (SD)	Mean (SD)		Mean (SD)	Mean (SD)	
Technology and Task Fitness	13.17 (2.0)	11.02 (2.9)	<0.001 *	12.49 (2.5)	12.09 (2.9)	0.118	12.09 (2.5)	12.55 (2.7)	0.06
Connectivity	13.06 (2.4)	10.98 (3.4)	<0.001 *	12.40 (2.9)	12.02 (3.2)	0.185	12.21 (2.9)	12.32 (3.1)	0.691
Communication	12.23 (3.2)	10.49 (3.8)	<0.001 *	11.67 (3.5)	11.39 (3.6)	0.413	11.25 (3.5)	11.89 (3.6)	0.08
Health Care	13.39 (1.9)	11.65 (3.1)	<0.001 *	12.84 (2.5)	12.52 (2.8)	0.196	12.67 (2.5)	12.77 (2.6)	0.684
Infotainment	11.68 (3.4)	10.35 (3.8)	<0.001 *	11.15 (3.6)	11.23 (3.6)	0.794	10.77 (3.6)	11.47 (3.5)	0.032 *
Fashionability	11.85 (3.2)	10.87 (3.5)	0.002 *	11.62 (3.2)	11.22 (3.7)	0.219	11.74 (3.1)	11.30 (3.5)	0.156
Wearability	12.52 (2.3)	11.26 (2.8)	<0.001 *	12.14 (2.5)	11.86 (2.8)	0.255	12.16 (2.4)	11.96 (2.8)	0.410
Subjective Norms	11.37 (3.6)	10.06 (3.7)	<0.001 *	10.92 (3.8)	10.79 (3.7)	0.714	10.58 (3.8)	11.09 (3.7)	0.139

Independent Sample t-test, * p-value < 0.05 is considered statistically significant.

4. Discussion

In this survey, we analyzed whether socio-demographic and usage-determining factors correlated with self-reported use of wearable devices for healthcare in a subset of the Indian population, mainly medical and engineering professionals. This study provides empirical support for the hypothesis that factors, drawn from the TAM and TTF models along with additionally considered variables determining the use, are positively correlated with the self-reported use of wearable devices for healthcare.

4.1. Theoretical Models to Study the Acceptance of Technology among Users

Various theories of behavior have been formulated giving rise to different models predicting human behavior. A prominent and well-studied model is the technology acceptance model (TAM). This is based on a major theory of human behavior, the theory of reasoned action (TRA). Another common model is the task-technology fitness (TTF) model used to study the congruence of new information systems with task requirements.

The theory of reasoned action (TRA) states a person's performance of a specified behavior is determined by their behavioral intention (BI) to perform it, which in turn is determined by the person's attitude (A) and subjective norm (SN) concerning the behavior. According to the TAM model, two main factors influence the acceptance of new technology by users—perceived usefulness (PU) and perceived ease of use (PEOU). PU has been defined as "the degree to which a person believes that using a particular system would enhance their job performance". PEOU has been defined as "the degree to which a person believes that using a particular system would be free from effort". Both influence attitude (A) toward using the technology which in turn influences BI, which determines the actual usage [17]. PU and PEOU are independently correlated with a higher frequency of self-reported use of new information technology by users [17–20]. TAM was modified to incorporate SN from TRA, such that SN acted as external variables that affected PU and PEOU. The TAM model has been widely used to study the adoption of disparate projects in the field of information technology [20–24]. The TTF model proposes that user performance is improved if there is a congruence of the technology with the task at hand. It suggests that technology will be used and will improve user performance only if tool functionality fits task requirements [25].

TAM focuses on attitudes behind technology adoption, while TTF focuses on the operational aspects. Subsequent research has tried to integrate the TTF and TAM models to better explain technology acceptance and proposed that TTF factors influence PU and PEOU [26].

4.2. Variables Studied and Analyzed during Our Survey

A recent study by Chang et al. (2016) proposed a technology acceptance model for wearable healthcare devices based on the TAM–TTF model and defined TTF factors for wearable healthcare devices as connectivity, communication, healthcare, and infotainment. This study also proposed that external factors such as subjective norms and device factors of wearability and fashionability influence BI [27].

Drawing from the TAM and TTF models, we constructed an abbreviated questionnaire, similar to the previously used and validated construct by Chang et al., consisting of three-question items, each to assess BI, PU, PEOU, and TTF using the Likert scale. Different from the original TTF construct, this model assessed a subjective sense of task and technology fitness, rather than focused objective factors. Factors for TTF for wearable devices were used as defined by previous studies. Connectivity describes the interaction between devices using Bluetooth or wireless network technology. Communication refers to the function of wearable devices that allow users to communicate with other users, such as by making phone calls, text messaging, etc. Healthcare refers to how wearable devices assist the user in managing their health. This was assessed using a subjective three-question item construct. Infotainment refers to factors such as the displayed information about heart rate and distance statistics to guide improvement or seek enjoyment and motivation as users engage in health-promoting behavior. Fashionability refers to fashion factors related to the design of the wearable device. This has been seen as weakly significant or correlated in comparison with the use of wearable devices for healthcare management purposes. Wearability refers to design factors of the wearable device related to form and fit, ease of wearability, access to the device, etc. Wearability is strongly positively correlated with task-technology fitness. Subjective norms are social factors, such as what an individual who is important to the user thinks about the device. Evidence for subjective norms affecting the use of new technology has been seen to be more significant for female users in the older age group in the early stages of use, but these findings are more important in mandatory usage settings. In the case of voluntary use such as wearables, subjective norm falls to how it affects attitude and behavioral intention [28].

Using these models of human behavior as a base, we have tried to construct our theoretical model to predict the adoption of wearable devices for healthcare and gauge the response of a sub-section of the Indian population, as explained above. We have not elicited what type of wearable devices were used by our respondents, or how they used them for managing health. However, wearable fitness trackers with pedometers and accelerometers are the most common wearable devices used for healthcare found on the market worldwide, while in India, the market is largely dominated by "hearables", smartwatches comprising the fastest growing device segment. This descriptive study largely applies to these devices [29,30].

4.3. Adoption of Wearable Healthcare Devices

Wearable devices and their specific use in healthcare management have been studied using various validated human behavior models, such as the TAM model, the successor UTAUT with protection motivation theory, and privacy calculus theory, which have recently evolved in the field to explain users' privacy concerns [31,32]. These studies have analyzed various factors that influence the adoption, continued use, frequency of use, and discontinuation of wearable devices. A recent national survey in the USA, studying the reception of wearable device technology in the western world, estimated that close to 30% of adults are using wearable healthcare devices. This nationwide survey also correlated socio-economic, demographic, health, and technology, self-efficacy attributes to the actual use of wearable devices [33].

In the present study, we found that subjective measurements of task-technology fitness (TTF) are strongly positively correlated with device factors of connectivity and healthcare, and moderately positively correlated with communication and infotainment. This reflects the users' perceptions that wearable devices are used mainly for healthcare, and for achieving health goals. The synchronization and connectivity of the wearable device to other devices are necessary for the ease of transfer of health data. Users/participants in the present study were not regularly using wearable healthcare devices for communication tasks such as making calls or messaging, as well as infotainment.

TTF measures were found to be strongly correlated with PU and PEOU. PU is strongly correlated with BI in previous studies using the TAM model on wearable devices and other technologies that are also in accordance with our study [20]. PEOU is less strongly correlated, which may be due to the moderating influence of PU on PEOU, which has been well described in the literature [17,25]. Wearability and subjective norm were moderately positively correlated with BI, and fashionability is less correlated with BI. This is similar to previous study observations, indicating that the wearability of the device, along with the perception of other people about wearable devices, significantly influences Behavioral intention to use them, though fashionability does not significantly affect it [27]. This shows the practicality aspect of users' intention that wearable devices are preferred for health care management rather than fashion sense.

All factors determining use were positively correlated with reported use, as respondents who were using wearable healthcare devices had higher mean scores than non-users. This gives an insight, that current users were happy with their product and hence were more motivated to use it. Males had a higher BI and PEOU than females. This follows a similar trend observed in the previous studies using TAM, and UTAUT models, which found females to have more difficulty learning how to operate new information technology and have lower scores of PEOU or higher scores of perceived difficulties [25–27]. The authors discussed the social context behind this, and they had hoped that this gap would reduce in the internet age. This may apply to India, but the Indian demographic may be more susceptible to lingering effects of gender disparity, opportunity, and exposure. Differences in other factors were non-significant. While wearable devices are more common among females, there is a mutually constitutive relationship between gender and technology, which in turn is adapted by technological transformations. It also means that societies with better gender equality also have a better digital economy.

Our study findings show an interesting trend where adults aged more than 25 years showed higher BI and infotainment. This may reflect changing perceptions around wearables for personal health management and fitness among older adults in India. This gives further reason for supporting the adoption of wearables as a cost-effective means of monitoring physical activity and maintaining general health.

The original TAM model pilot study used a 10-question item construct to measure PU and PEOU. This model was abbreviated in the present study to three questions per domain. The original UTAUT study used measures of performance expectancy, effort expectancy, and social influence that act on behavioral intention, which determines usage. Performance expectancy is a similar construct to PU, and effort expectancy to PEOU in TAM. Social norms in TAM2 have been seen to be similar to social influence in UTAUT. The study included three-question items similar to those used in the final UTAUT question construct, which was formulated to ensure the highest object loading and degrees of freedom according to psychometric theories, which may compromise content validity due to insufficient representation of the content [26,27].

Privacy remains a major point of concern for consumers interested in wearable healthcare devices. In particular, the release of personal information and data for analysis carries the risk of dissemination, leak, and unauthorized use [34–36]. A distinct challenge that arises in India is the heterogeneity in the availability and quality of devices. Consumer devices are not subjected to regulatory frameworks and rigorous testing that medical devices typically undergo, which poses concerns about the validity of device recordings and data security concerns. The worldwide wearable devices market ballooned in 2014 and has since resulted in a plethora of device types with different sensors, software, and design that have entered the Indian market as well. This adds additional factors that contribute to the acceptance and usage of devices, including the type and accuracy of sensors, the complexity of the user interface, and brand value perception. Only a few brands have been used and validated in formal research studies. Researchers have developed a comprehensive device evaluation tool that may be used to guide future regulatory policies [37]. Another challenge is the high attrition rate and fall in the usage of wearable devices over time. A 2016 survey found that 30% of users of a popular brand name fitness tracker discontinue use within 6 months [38]. A 2019 study found that 20% of users abandoned their devices, with the most common reasons cited to be related to data literacy, or device comfort [39]. Age and limited technology literacy, with issues related to perceived measurement inaccuracy, have been seen to be major factors for device abandonment, and pose a significant challenge to behavioral change and long-term healthcare management goals [40,41]. Behavioral change techniques (BCT) such as just-in-time adaptive interventions, for example, motivational mobile messages accompanying device notifications and gamification, have been seen to be effective at increasing physical activity and may help solidify behavioral changes [42,43].

4.4. Limitations

The survey was primarily circulated among professionals interested in technology and personal healthcare technology, and this may be a source of sampling bias. Since we only examined a narrow subset of the population in the context of India, the generalizability and interpretation cannot be extrapolated to other contexts as in different countries or different social backgrounds. Although we compared differences across gender and age groups, we did not look into and compare differences across income groups. Moreover, all questionnaire responses are self-reported, and reflect subjective perceptions about factors and therefore may be subject to interpretation bias by participants. This is a questionnaire survey, hence cannot elicit development, use, or loss to attrition of wearable healthcare devices use, which has been elucidated in multiple previous studies [23,24]. Hence, conducting longitudinal studies will better address the issue of factors determining long-term use. Our model is constructed based on the TAM and TTF models. Although aspects of privacy calculus theory such as hedonic motivation, performance expectancy, etc. can be equated to similar measures used in TAM and TTF, it does not include the privacy calculus model, which also addresses concerns regarding personal health data security and privacy.

5. Conclusions

The use of wearable healthcare device usage has skyrocketed in India over the past few years. This is important for the medicine and healthcare industry because wearable devices play an important role in monitoring and preventing chronic diseases to a certain level. In a developing country such as India, diseases and hospitalization make a major impact on the financial status of the family, in turn affecting their quality of life. The present study helps in filling the significant research gap of studies looking at the adoption and acceptance of wearable devices in the context of a low-middle-income country.

Supplementary Materials: The following supporting information can be downloaded at: https://www.mdpi.com/article/10.3390/jcm11237019/s1. Use of Wearable Health Care Devices by Adults in Managing Personal Health—A Questionnaire.

Author Contributions: Conceptualization, V.P., D.K.S., N.N. and B.M.Z.H.; methodology, B.M.Z.H., M.J.S., S.I., K.S. and G.C.; software, D.K.S., N.N., A.K., A.S. and R.P.; investigation, V.P. and D.K.S.; resources, M.J.S., S.I. and K.S.; data curation, M.J.S., S.I., K.S. and D.K.S.; writing—original draft preparation, V.P., D.K.S., K.S., G.C. and A.K.; writing—review and editing, N.N., R.P., P.C. and B.K.S.; visualization, R.P. and P.C.; project administration, N.N., B.M.Z.H. and B.K.S. All authors have read and agreed to the published version of the manuscript.

Funding: This research has not received external funding.

Institutional Review Board Statement: This research was conducted with permission from the Institutional Ethics Committee. Data acquisition and analysis were performed with the protocols approved by the Institutional Ethical committee (ethical approval number FMIEC-94/2021). Informed consent was obtained from all the participants before the study. All procedures performed in this study involving human participants were in accordance with the ethical standards of the institutional and/or national research committee and with the 1964 Helsinki declaration and its later amendments or comparable ethical standards.

Informed Consent Statement: All participants provided informed consent to participate in the survey and use their data for scientific purposes.

Data Availability Statement: All data and material collected are presented in the manuscript. Clarification on any matter can be made through the corresponding author.

Conflicts of Interest: The authors declare no conflict of interest.

References

1. Lu, L.; Zhang, J.; Xie, Y.; Gao, F.; Xu, S.; Wu, X.; Ye, Z. Wearable Health Devices in Health Care: Narrative Systematic Review. *JMIR mHealth uHealth* **2020**, *8*, e18907. [CrossRef] [PubMed]
2. Mills, M. Hearing aids and the history of electronics miniaturization. *IEEE Ann. Hist. Comput.* **2011**, *33*, 24–45. [CrossRef]
3. Oswald, A. *At the Heart of the Invention: The development of the Holter Monitor*; National Museum of American History: Washington, DC, USA, 2014; Volume 8.
4. Ioannou, K.; Ignaszewski, M.; Macdonald, I. Ambulatory electrocardiography: The contribution of Norman Jefferis Holter. *BC Med. J.* **2014**, *56*, 86–89.
5. Kvedar, J.; Coye, M.J.; Everett, W. Connected Health: A Review of Technologies and Strategies to Improve Patient Care with Telemedicine and Telehealth. *Health Aff.* **2014**, *33*, 194–199. [CrossRef] [PubMed]
6. Ray, P.P.; Dash, D.; De, D. A Systematic Review of Wearable Systems for Cancer Detection: Current State and Challenges. *J. Med. Syst.* **2017**, *41*, 180. [CrossRef] [PubMed]
7. Li, X.; Dunn, J.; Salins, D.; Zhou, G.; Zhou, W.; Rose, S.M.S.-F.; Perelman, D.; Colbert, E.; Runge, R.; Rego, S.; et al. Digital Health: Tracking Physiomes and Activity Using Wearable Biosensors Reveals Useful Health-Related Information. *PLoS Biol.* **2017**, *15*, e2001402. [CrossRef] [PubMed]
8. Lapointe, J.; Bécotte-Boutin, H.-S.; Gagnon, S.; Levasseur, S.; Labranche, P.; D'Auteuil, M.; Abdellatif, M.; Li, M.-J.; Vallée, R. Smartphone Screen Integrated Optical Breathalyzer. *Sensors* **2021**, *21*, 4076. [CrossRef]
9. Pyrkov, T.V.; Slipensky, K.; Barg, M.; Kondrashin, A.; Zhurov, B.; Zenin, A.; Pyatnitskiy, M.; Menshikov, L.; Markov, S.; Fedichev, P.O. Extracting biological age from biomedical data via deep learning: Too much of a good thing? *Sci. Rep.* **2018**, *8*, 5210. [CrossRef]
10. Moon, J.H.; Kang, M.-K.; Choi, C.-E.; Min, J.; Lee, H.-Y.; Lim, S. Validation of a wearable cuff-less wristwatch-type blood pressure monitoring device. *Sci. Rep.* **2020**, *10*, 19015. [CrossRef] [PubMed]
11. Franssen, W.; Franssen, G.H.L.M.; Spaas, J.; Solmi, F.; Eijnde, B.O. Can consumer wearable activity tracker-based interventions improve physical activity and cardiometabolic health in patients with chronic diseases? A systematic review and meta-analysis of randomised controlled trials. *Int. J. Behav. Nutr. Phys. Act.* **2020**, *17*, 57. [CrossRef]
12. Yen, H.-Y. Smart wearable devices as a psychological intervention for healthy lifestyle and quality of life: A randomized controlled trial. *Qual. Life Res.* **2021**, *30*, 791–802. [CrossRef] [PubMed]
13. Saini, G.; Budhwar, V.; Choudhary, M. Review on people's trust on home use medical devices during COVID-19 pandemic in India. *Health Technol.* **2022**, *12*, 527–546. [CrossRef] [PubMed]
14. Koo, S.H. Consumer Differences in the United States and India on Wearable Trackers. *Fam. Consum. Sci. Res. J.* **2017**, *46*, 40–56. [CrossRef]
15. Pandey, S.; Chawla, D.; Puri, S.; Jeong, L.S. Acceptance of wearable fitness devices in developing countries: Exploring the country and gender-specific differences. *J. Asia Bus. Stud.* **2021**, *16*, 676–692. [CrossRef]
16. Devine, J.K.; Schwartz, L.P.; Choynowski, J.; Hursh, S.R. Expert Demand for Consumer Sleep Technology Features and Wearable Devices: A Case Study. *IoT* **2022**, *3*, 315–331. [CrossRef]
17. Jeong, J.-Y.; Roh, T.-W. The Intention of Using Wearable Devices: Based on Modified Technology Acceptance Model. *J. Digit. Converg.* **2017**, *15*, 205–212. [CrossRef]
18. Adams, D.A.; Nelson, R.R.; Todd, P.A. Perceived Usefulness, Ease of Use, and Usage of Information Technology: A Replication. *MIS Q.* **1992**, *16*, 227–247. [CrossRef]
19. Szajna, B. Software Evaluation and Choice: Predictive Validation of the Technology Acceptance Instrument. *MIS Q.* **1994**, *18*, 319. [CrossRef]
20. Rahimi, B.; Nadri, H.; Afshar, H.L.; Timpka, T. A Systematic Review of the Technology Acceptance Model in Health Informatics. *Appl. Clin. Inform.* **2018**, *9*, 604–634. [CrossRef]

21. Verdru, J.; Van Paesschen, W. Wearable seizure detection devices in refractory epilepsy. *Acta Neurol. Belg.* **2020**, *120*, 1271–1281. [CrossRef]
22. Nelson, B.W.; Allen, N.B. Accuracy of Consumer Wearable Heart Rate Measurement During an Ecologically Valid 24-Hour Period: Intraindividual Validation Study. *JMIR mHealth uHealth* **2019**, *7*, e10828. [CrossRef]
23. Ocagli, H.; Lorenzoni, G.; Lanera, C.; Schiavo, A.; D'Angelo, L.; Di Liberti, A.; Besola, L.; Cibin, G.; Martinato, M.; Azzolina, D.; et al. Monitoring Patients Reported Outcomes after Valve Replacement Using Wearable Devices: Insights on Feasibility and Capability Study: Feasibility Results. *Int. J. Environ. Res. Public Health* **2021**, *18*, 7171. [CrossRef] [PubMed]
24. Rodriguez-León, C.; Villalonga, C.; Munoz-Torres, M.; Ruiz, J.R.; Banos, O. Mobile and wearable technology for the monitoring of diabetes-related parameters: Systematic review. *JMIR mHealth and uHealth* **2021**, *9*, e25138. [CrossRef] [PubMed]
25. Goodhue, D.L.; Thompson, R.L. Task-Technology Fit and Individual Performance. *MIS Q.* **1995**, *19*, 213–236. [CrossRef]
26. Dishaw, M.T.; Strong, D.M. Extending the technology acceptance model with task–technology fit constructs. *Inf. Manag.* **1999**, *36*, 9–21. [CrossRef]
27. Chang, H.S.; Lee, S.C.; Ji, Y.G. Wearable device adoption model with TAM and TTF. *Int. J. Mob. Commun.* **2016**, *14*, 518. [CrossRef]
28. Venkatesh, V.; Morris, M.G.; Davis, G.B.; Davis, F.D. User acceptance of information technology: Toward a unified view. *MIS Q.* **2003**, *27*, 425–478. [CrossRef]
29. Bove, L.A. Increasing Patient Engagement Through the Use of Wearable Technology. *J. Nurse Pract.* **2019**, *15*, 535–539. [CrossRef]
30. Bhargava, S.; Gupta, P. Boat: The Indian startup scripts a revolutionizing growth strategy. *Emerald Emerg. Mark. Case Stud.* **2022**, *12*, 1–40. [CrossRef]
31. Gao, Y.; Li, H.; Luo, Y. An empirical study of wearable technology acceptance in healthcare. *Ind. Manag. Data Syst.* **2015**, *115*, 1704–1723. [CrossRef]
32. Al-Maroof, R.S.; Alhumaid, K.; Alhamad, A.Q.; Aburayya, A.; Salloum, S. User Acceptance of Smart Watch for Medical Purposes: An Empirical Study. *Future Internet* **2021**, *13*, 127. [CrossRef]
33. Chandrasekaran, R.; Katthula, V.; Moustakas, E. Patterns of Use and Key Predictors for the Use of Wearable Health Care Devices by US Adults: Insights from a National Survey. *J. Med. Internet Res.* **2020**, *22*, e22443. [CrossRef] [PubMed]
34. Cheatham, S.W.; Stull, K.R.; Fantigrassi, M.; Motel, I. The efficacy of wearable activity tracking technology as part of a weight loss program: A systematic review. *J. Sports Med. Phys. Fit.* **2018**, *58*, 534–548. [CrossRef] [PubMed]
35. Fawcett, E.; Van Velthoven, M.H.; Meinert, E. Long-Term Weight Management Using Wearable Technology in Overweight and Obese Adults: Systematic Review. *JMIR mHealth uHealth* **2020**, *8*, e13461. [CrossRef] [PubMed]
36. Maddison, R.; Cartledge, S.; Rogerson, M.; Goedhart, N.S.; Singh, T.R.; Neil, C.; Phung, D.; Ball, K. Usefulness of Wearable Cameras as a Tool to Enhance Chronic Disease Self-Management: Scoping Review. *JMIR mHealth uHealth* **2019**, *7*, e10371. [CrossRef]
37. Bayoumy, K.; Gaber, M.; Elshafeey, A.; Mhaimeed, O.; Dineen, E.H.; Marvel, F.A.; Martin, S.S.; Muse, E.D.; Turakhia, M.P.; Tarakji, K.G.; et al. Smart wearable devices in cardiovascular care: Where we are and how to move forward. *Nat. Rev. Cardiol.* **2021**, *18*, 581–599. [CrossRef]
38. Gartner Survey Shows Wearable Devices Need to Be More Useful [Internet]. Available online: https://www.gartner.com/en/newsroom/press-releases/2016-12-07-gartner-survey-shows-wearable-devices-need-to-be-more-useful (accessed on 19 June 2022).
39. Jarusriboonchai, P.; Häkkilä, J. Customisable wearables: Exploring the design space of wearable technology. In Proceedings of the 18th International Conference on Mobile and Ubiquitous Multimedia 2019, Pisa, Italy, 26–29 November 2019; pp. 1–9.
40. Steinert, A.; Haesner, M.; Steinhagen-Thiessen, E. Activity-tracking devices for older adults: Comparison and preferences. *Univers. Access Inf. Soc.* **2018**, *17*, 411–419. [CrossRef]
41. Kononova, A.; Li, L.; Kamp, K.; Bowen, M.; Rikard, R.V.; Cotten, S.; Peng, W. The Use of Wearable Activity Trackers among Older Adults: Focus Group Study of Tracker Perceptions, Motivators, and Barriers in the Maintenance Stage of Behavior Change. *JMIR mHealth uHealth* **2019**, *7*, e9832. [CrossRef]
42. Martin, S.S.; Feldman, D.I.; Blumenthal, R.S.; Jones, S.R.; Post, W.S.; McKibben, R.A.; Michos, E.D.; Ndumele, C.E.; Ratchford, E.V.; Coresh, J.; et al. mActive: A randomized clinical trial of an automated mHealth intervention for physical activity promotion. *J. Am. Heart Assoc.* **2015**, *4*, e002239. [CrossRef]
43. Patel, M.S.; Benjamin, E.J.; Volpp, K.G.; Fox, C.S.; Small, D.S.; Massaro, J.M.; Lee, J.J.; Hilbert, V.; Valentino, M.; Taylor, D.H.; et al. Effect of a game-based intervention designed to enhance social incentives to increase physical activity among families: The BE FIT randomized clinical trial. *JAMA Intern. Med.* **2017**, *177*, 1586–1593. [CrossRef]

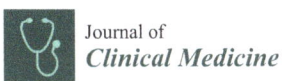

Article

Totally X-ray-Free Ultrasound-Guided Mini-Percutaneous Nephrolithotomy in Galdakao-Modified Supine Valdivia Position: A Novel Combined Surgery

Yi-Yang Liu [1,2], Yen-Ta Chen [1], Hao-Lun Luo [1], Yuan-Chi Shen [1], Chien-Hsu Chen [1], Yao-Chi Chuang [1], Ko-Wei Huang [2] and Hung-Jen Wang [1,*]

[1] Department of Urology, Kaohsiung Chang Gung Memorial Hospital and Chang Gung University College of Medicine, Kaohsiung 83301, Taiwan
[2] Department of Electrical Engineering, National Kaohsiung University of Science and Technology, Kaohsiung 80778, Taiwan
* Correspondence: hujewang@gmail.com

Abstract: We introduced a novel surgery that combines ultrasound guidance, miniaturization and Galdakao-modified supine Valdivia (GMSV) position in percutaneous nephrolithotomy (PCNL) and evaluated the safety and efficacy. This retrospective, single-center study retrospectively reviewed 150 patients who underwent ultrasound-guided mini-PCNL in the GMSV position from November 2019 to March 2022. All perioperative parameters were collected. Stone-free status was defined as no residual stones or clinically insignificant residual fragments (CIRF) <0.4 cm on postoperative day one. Among the 150 patients, the mean age was 56.96 years. The mean stone size was 3.19 cm (427 mm^2). The mean S.T.O.N.E. score was 7.61, including 36 patients (24%) with scores ≥9. The mean operative time was 66.22 min, and the success rate of renal access creation in the first attempt was 88.7%. One hundred and forty (93.3%) patients were stone free. The mean decrease in Hemoglobin was 1.04 g/dL, and no patient needed a blood transfusion. Complications included transient hematuria (n = 13, 8.7%), bladder blood clot retention (n = 2, 1.3%), fever (n = 15, 10%) and sepsis (n = 2, 1.3%). Totally X-ray-free ultrasound-guided mini-PCNL in the GMSV position is feasible, safe and effective for patients with upper urinary tract stones, indicating the synergistic and complementary effects of the three novel techniques.

Keywords: mini-PCNL; ultrasound guidance; GMSV position

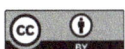

1. Introduction

Percutaneous nephrolithotomy (PCNL) was first introduced in 1976 [1], and over the years, it has become the gold standard of surgical treatment for renal stones larger than 2 cm [2]. Conventionally, PCNL was performed via a larger percutaneous nephrostomy (PCN) tract (≥22 French) [3], under fluoroscopic guidance, with patients in the prone position. Gradually, three novel techniques have been developed and widely accepted. First, ultrasound-guided PCNL reduces or even eliminates radiation exposure by fluoroscopy [4]. Moreover, mini-PCNL with miniaturization of the PCN tract (<22 French) [3] decreases renal trauma compared to standard PCNL [5]. Moreover, mini-PCNL demonstrated non-inferior surgical outcomes to standard PCNL for 2- to 4-cm-sized renal stones [6]. Finally, the Galdakao-modified supine Valdivia (GMSV) position facilitates simultaneous bidirectional endourological procedures rather than using the prone position [7].

Nevertheless, each of these three techniques also has its own weak points. First, it is not easy to monitor the process of PCN tract dilation using ultrasound guidance [8]. In addition, mini-PCNL is associated with lower lithotripsy efficiency and longer operative time [9]. Finally, the GMSV position may lead to renal displacement during PCN tract dilation and a narrow operating space during lithotripsy [10]. Fortunately, these three techniques have complementary advantages when they are combined. In the GMSV position, retrograde semi-rigid ureteroscopic assistance can be used to increase the safety of the puncture and dilation process [11]. In addition, the GMSV position improves the efficiency of mini-PCNL lithotripsy by the horizontal or downward axis of the Amplatz-type renal sheath [10]. Moreover, the GMSV position avoids repositioning from the lithotomy position to the prone position and, therefore, decreases the total operative time [12]. Mini-PCNL makes up for the insufficient operating space in the GMSV position [13]. Finally, ultrasound guidance facilitates PCNL in the supine position, including in the GMSV position [8].

Based on these complementary properties, we combined these three techniques for PCNL. To the best of our knowledge, studies of PCNL using the three combined techniques are limited. Therefore, we conducted a retrospective, single-center study to evaluate the outcomes of patients undergoing totally X-ray-free ultrasound-guided mini-PCNL in the GMSV position.

2. Materials and Methods

2.1. Study Design and Sample

This retrospective cohort study retrospectively reviewed the data of consecutive patients with upper urinary tract stone disease who had undergone one-step totally X-ray-free ultrasound-guided single-tract mini-PCNL in the GMSV position from November 2019 to March 2022 at Kaohsiung Chang Gung Memorial Hospital. Patients with age <18 years old, pregnancy, radiolucent stone, abnormal upper urinary tract anatomy (including horseshoe kidney, renal duplication, ureteropelvic junction obstruction, or ureteral stricture), preoperative severe urinary tract infection such as acute pyelonephritis or urosepsis, bleeding tendency, concurrent malignancy, multiple-tract PCNL, concurrent bilateral urinary tract endoscopic stone surgery, incomplete perioperative data or loss of follow-up were excluded. Finally, a total of 150 patients were included in the study.

2.2. Ethical Considerations

The protocol of the present study was approved by the Institutional Review Board of Kaohsiung Chang Gung Memorial Hospital (No. 202201106B0). Due to the retrospective study design, the IRB waived informed consent of the included patients.

2.3. Surgical Procedure and Statistical Analysis

All PCNL operations were performed by the same urologist (Dr. Yi Yang Liu). All included patients received basic preoperative examination, including non-contrast computed tomography (NCCT) of abdomen for image survey. The S.T.O.N.E. nephrolithotomy score (a graded system to predict patients' stone-free status) was calculated according to NCCT findings [14]. Moreover, preoperative urinary culture was collected. If the result was positive, we would use intravenous antibiotics for the pathogen during the perioperative period. Otherwise, prophylactic antibiotics would be administered to the patients 30 min before the operation and kept for 24 h after the operation.

The patient was placed in the GMSV position under general anesthesia [7]. Ipsilateral 4 or 5 French ureteral catheterization was performed initially to create artificial hydronephrosis by manual ureteral catheter injection of 0.9% sodium chloride solution. Then, an ultrasound-guided (BK5000, BK Medical, Herlev, Denmark) 18-gauge needle transpapillary puncture toward the target renal calyx was performed with the assistance of a puncture frame. The needle tip in the renal collecting system was confirmed by the urine efflux from the puncture needle sheath, and the puncture depth was then measured. Subsequently, a 0.035-inch J-tip guidewire was indwelled into the puncture needle sheath, and a 0.6 cm skin incision was made. Sequentially, both 8 and 10 French fascial dilators were followed by the puncture depth. Finally, an 18 French Ultraxx™ Nephrostomy Balloon Catheter (Cook Medical, Bloomington, IN, USA) was indwelled and inflated with 0.9% sodium chloride solution under the pressure of 20 atm for 3 min, and an 18 French Amplatz-type renal sheath was introduced to create the renal access. The dilation procedures were monitored by real-time ultrasound in as much detail as possible [15].

After creating the renal access, a 12 French Miniature Nephroscope (Richard Wolf, Knittlingen, Germany) and Holmium laser (Auriga XL 50 Watt, Boston Scientific, Boston, MA, USA) were used for stone fragmentation. The broken stone chips were washed out by low-pressure irrigation with 0.9% sodium chloride solution continuous irrigation from the mere height of 70 cm above the operating table. No irrigation pump or negative pressure suction device was used. Residual stones were checked by the nephroscope and ultrasound. Finally, a 4.7 or 6 French Double J stent was indwelled by the nephroscope. Either no catheter or a 14 French percutaneous nephrostomy balloon catheter was installed with 1 to 3 cc distilled water, depending on the surgeon's decision. Simultaneously, retrograde semi-rigid ureteroscopy may be performed if indicated (e.g., failed artificial hydronephrosis creation by ureteral catheterization, confirmation of the guidewire or puncture needle tip in collecting system, residual stone in upper ureter or upper calyx, or failed antegrade Double J stenting). Operative time was defined as the time from ureteral catheterization to removal of the Amplatz sheath or the placement of the percutaneous nephrostomy balloon catheter.

Stone fragments were sent for analysis postoperatively. Blood examination and kidney ureter bladder (KUB) plain X-ray were performed on postoperative day one. Stone-free status was defined as no residual stone or clinically insignificant residual fragment (CIRF) <0.4 cm in KUB on postoperative day one. All perioperative data and events associated with postoperative surgical complications within one month were recorded. All descriptive statistics were analyzed using IBM SPSS version 21.0 Software (IBM, Armonk, NY, USA).

3. Results

The patients' characteristics are listed in Table 1. Among the 150 patients, the mean age was 56.96 years, including 90 male patients and 60 female patients. Ninety-two patients underwent left-side PCNL. The mean body mass index (BMI) was 26 kg/m^2, and 16.7% of the patients were obese (BMI > 30 kg/m^2). The mean stone size and burden were 3.19 cm and 427 mm^2, respectively. Twenty-two patients (14.7%) had staghorn stones, and 38 patients (25.3%) had both renal and upper ureteral stones. Mean stone density was 1199 Hounsfield units. Seventy percent of the patients have moderate to severe hydronephrosis. Twelve patients (8%) have history of percutaneous nephrolithotomy or open nephrolithotomy. High stone complexity (S.T.O.N.E. score ≥ 9) was noted in 36 patients (24%). The majority of patients (75.3%) belong to American Society of Anesthesiologists (ASA) classification 1 or 2. Preoperative mean hemoglobin (14.05 g/dL), mean creatinine (1.04 mg/dL), mean estimated glomerular filtration rate (eGFR) (74.3 mL/min/1.73 m^2) and mean visual analog scale (VAS) for pain (0.35) were basically normal. In addition, 44 patients (29.3%) had positive urine cultures and underwent specific antibiotics treatment during the all-perioperative period.

Table 2 demonstrates the intraoperative parameters. The mean operative time was 66.22 min. Subcostal (93.3%) and middle calyceal (56.7%) punctures were used most frequently. The mean puncture depth was 8.84 cm. Thirty patients (20%) underwent non-hydronephrotic calyceal puncture with difficulty. However, the success rate of renal access creation on the first attempt was 88.7%. Retrograde semi-rigid ureteroscopic assistance was performed in 49 patients (32.7%). Tubeless procedures were performed in 21 patients (14%).

Table 1. Patients' characteristics.

Variables	(n = 150)
Age, years (mean ± SD)	56.96 ± 12.45
Gender (Male/Female)	90/60
Laterality (Left/Right)	92/58
Body mass index, kg/m² (mean ± SD)	26.00 ± 4.27
Obesity (Body mass index > 30 kg/m²), n (%)	25 (16.7%)
Total stone size, cm (mean ± SD)	3.19 ± 1.67
Total stone burden, mm² (mean ± SD)	427 ± 360
Stone number	
Single, n (%)	42 (28.0%)
Multiple, n (%)	86 (57.3%)
Staghorn stone, n (%)	22 (14.7%)
Stone location	
Kidney, n (%)	90 (60.0%)
Upper ureter, n (%)	22 (14.7%)
Kidney and upper ureter, n (%)	38 (25.3%)
Stone density, Hounsfield unit (mean ± SD)	1199.1 ± 309.2
S.T.O.N.E. Score (mean ± SD)	7.61 ± 1.36
S.T.O.N.E. Score ≥ 9, n (%)	36 (24.0%)
Preoperative hydronephrosis	
None, n (%)	32 (21.3%)
Mild, n (%)	13 (8.7%)
Moderate, n (%)	78 (52.0%)
Severe, n (%)	27 (18.0%)
Previous surgery	
ESWL or URSM or RIRS, n (%)	57 (38.0%)
PCNL or open surgery, n (%)	12 (8.0%)
ASA classification	
1, n (%)	5 (3.3%)
2, n (%)	108 (72.0%)
3, n (%)	36 (24.0%)
4, n (%)	1 (0.7%)
Preoperative Hemoglobin, g/dL (mean ± SD)	14.05 ± 1.64
Preoperative Creatinine, mg/dL (mean ± SD)	1.04 ± 0.41
Preoperative eGFR (MDRD), mL/min/1.73 m² (mean ± SD)	74.30 ± 24.23
Preoperative positive urine culture, n (%)	44 (29.3%)
Preoperative pain scale, visual analog scale (mean ± SD)	0.35 ± 0.83

SD = standard deviation; ESWL = extracorporeal shock wave lithotripsy; URSM = ureteroscopic stone manipulation; RIRS = retrograde intrarenal surgery; PCNL = percutaneous nephrolithotomy; ASA = American Society of Anesthesiologists; eGFR = estimated glomerular filtration rate; MDRD = modification of diet in renal disease.

Table 2. Intraoperative parameters.

Parameters	(n = 150)
Operative time, min (mean ± SD)	66.22 ± 36.54
Target calyx	
Upper, n (%)	14 (9.3%)
Middle, n (%)	85 (56.7%)
Lower, n (%)	51 (34.0%)
Puncture site	
11th intercostal space, n (%)	10 (6.7%)
Subcostal area, n (%)	140 (93.3%)
Non-hydronephrotic calyceal puncture, n (%)	30 (20.0%)
Success of renal access creation in the first attempt, n (%)	133 (88.7%)
Puncture depth, cm (mean ± SD)	8.84 ± 1.90
Retrograde semi-rigid ureteroscopic assistance, n (%)	49 (32.7%)
Tubeless, n (%)	21 (14.0%)

SD = standard deviation.

Postoperative outcomes are shown in Table 3. The mean hospital stay was 3.73 days, and immediate stone-free rate was 93.3% (140 patients). The mean reduction in hemoglobin was 1.04 g/dL. Compared to preoperative status, the mean postoperative eGFR was increased by 10.63 mL/min/1.73 m². The mean postoperative VAS for pain was 2.99. Only 30 patients (20%) had postoperative VAS for pain ≥4 and needed postoperative intravenous analgesic agents for pain control. For stone analysis, 109 patients (72.7%) had calcium oxalate as the predominant stone. Regarding postoperative infection, 15 patients (10%) experienced fever >38 °C postoperatively. The fever was transient and subsided after antipyretic treatment in most patients. Only two patients (1.3%) had urosepsis but recovered soon without septic shock after broad-spectrum antibiotics treatment. In terms of hemorrhagic complications, 13 patients (8.7%) had transient gross hematuria that subsided spontaneously. Bladder blood clot retention was noted in two patients (1.3%) who underwent cystoscopic blood clot evacuation under general anesthesia. No blood transfusions, radiological interventions or nephrectomy for bleeding control were needed. Moreover, no intensive care unit transferation, chest or abdominal organ injury or mortality was noted. To sum up, the majority of the complications were classified as Clavien–Dindo Grade I. The incidence of Clavien–Dindo grade II and grade IIIb complications were only 1.3% and 1.3%, respectively.

Table 3. Postoperative outcomes.

Variables		(n = 150)
Hospital stay, days (mean ± SD)		3.73 ± 1.59
Stone-free status, n (%)		140 (93.3%)
Postoperative Hemoglobin, g/dL (mean ± SD)		13.01 ± 1.70
Hemoglobin drop, g/dL (mean ± SD)		1.04 ± 1.10
Postoperative Creatinine, mg/dL (mean ± SD)		0.92 ± 0.34
Postoperative eGFR (MDRD), mL/min/1.73 m² (mean ± SD)		85.26 ± 27.47
Change of eGFR (MDRD), mL/min/1.73 m² (mean ± SD)		10.63 ± 18.27
Postoperative pain scale, visual analog scale (mean ± SD)		2.99 ± 1.50
Stone analysis		
	Calcium oxalate predominant, n (%)	109 (72.7%)
	Calcium phosphate predominant, n (%)	41 (27.3%)
Complications classified by Clavien–Dindo classification		
Grade I		
	Fever > 38 °C, n (%)	15 (10.0%)
	Transient gross hematuria, n (%)	13 (8.7%)
	Postoperative pain scale ≥ 4, n (%)	30 (20.0%)
Grade II		
	Sepsis, n (%)	2 (1.3%)
Grade IIIb		
	Bladder blood clot retention, n (%)	2 (1.3%)

SD = standard deviation; eGFR = estimated glomerular filtration rate; MDRD = modification of diet in renal disease.

4. Discussion

The results have revealed that totally X-ray-free ultrasound-guided mini-PCNL in the GMSV position is feasible with safety and efficacy. The mean operative time was about one hour, and the majority of cases had successful renal access creation on the first attempt. Postoperative outcomes showed that the majority of patients were stone free, and no major complication was noted. In the following discussion, we will analyze the detailed advantages through the whole process of PCNL. Figure 1 summarizes the three core techniques we used in the study and their effects on surgical outcomes.

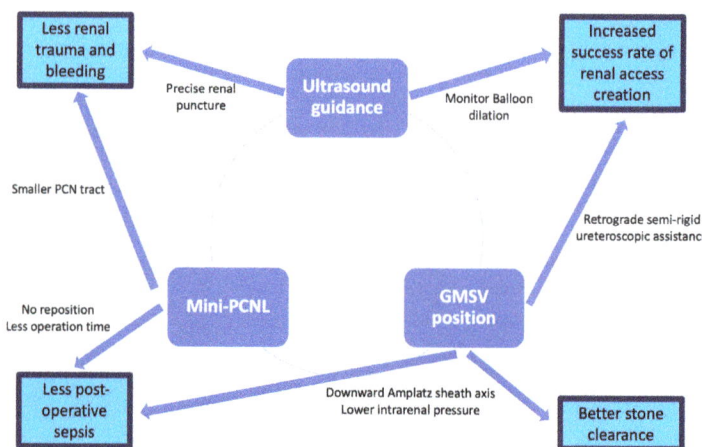

Figure 1. Three core techniques and their effects on surgical outcomes.

The GMSV position, which is the combination of the oblique supine position and lithotomy position, simultaneously facilitates bidirectional endourological procedures without repositioning and saves significant operative time [7]. There is also no chest or abdominal compression in the GMSV position, which enables anesthesiologists to easily monitor and control each patient's condition intraoperatively. Moreover, urologists can be seated with better ergonomics during the surgery [10]. Therefore, we can use the GMSV position throughout the procedures of PCNL with safety and efficacy.

In percutaneous renal calyceal puncture, ultrasound guidance requires no radiation exposure and provides easy identification of the posterior calyx and perirenal adjacent organs. In the present case series, no patient experienced pleura or perirenal organ injury. In addition, arterial puncture can be avoided under doppler mode ultrasound [8]. Hence, the risk of hemorrhagic complications is also decreased. The GMSV position also aids the puncture procedure because it allows retrograde semi-rigid ureteroscopic assistance to enhance retrograde ureteral irrigation when artificial hydronephrosis cannot be created by the ureteral catheter. Surgeons may also see the puncture needle tip or guidewire directly in the renal pelvis or ureter using the retrograde semi-rigid ureteroscope to ensure a successful renal puncture.

The rest part of renal access creation, including PCN tract dilation and Amplatz-type renal sheath setup, is a critical step before lithotripsy. Under the GMSV position, renal mobility is typically obvious because of the absence of abdominal compression, and it may lead to a shorter dilation or guidewire slippage and then failure of renal access creation [10]. To reduce renal mobility, we used skills such as coordinated abdominal counterpressure and brief apnea in maximal inspiration. Additionally, the use of the balloon dilator reduces the number of times of repetitive and sequential PCN tract dilation. Moreover, balloon dilation can be monitored under ultrasound during inflation [15]. Moreover, retrograde semi-rigid ureteroscopic assistance has been used for difficult cases by setting up a through-and-through guidewire to secure the subsequent renal access creation procedures [11]. In the present study, 20% of patients underwent non-hydronephrotic calyceal puncture. Even so, the success rate of renal access creation in the first attempt was still 88.7%. This result is comparable with that of another study in terms of ultrasound-guided conventional PCNL with balloon dilation in the prone position performed by very experienced urologists (88.4%) [15]. In other words, renal access creation by ultrasound-guided mini-PCNL in the GMSV position is shown to be feasible with a high success rate in the first attempt.

The vacuum cleaner effect of lithotripsy during mini-PCNL is the basic mechanism for stone fragment removal [16]. Conventionally, mini-PCNL often needs an irrigation pump with high irrigation pressure (150 to 250 mmHg) to effectively remove stone fragments [17].

In the GMSV position, the axis of the Amplatz-type renal sheath is horizontal or slightly inclined downward toward the ground. There is no doubt that this will enhance the vacuum cleaner effect compared to the prone position [10]. In the present study, just gravity irrigation with low irrigation pressure (70 cm H_2O) was used for stone fragment removal, and there was no need for the irrigation pump. Additionally, compared to the standard PCNL, the mini-PCNL allows greater exploration from the single calyx to most of the desired locations in the renal collecting system without placing excessive torque on the renal parenchyma [13]. This advantage of the mini-PCNL compensates for the restricted working space and limited instrument movement through the longer PCN tract in the GMSV position [10]. Moreover, if residual fragments are found in the upper ureter or upper calyx, retrograde semi-rigid ureteroscopy is also readily available for lithotripsy. Although 24% of patients in the present study had complex renal stones with S.T.O.N.E. nephrolithotomy scores ≥9, the overall stone-free rate was still 93.3%, which was comparable with other studies of mini-PCNL (ranging from 75.0% to 95.1%) [18] or the pooled data from the latest meta-analysis (85.1%) [19].

In the literature review, Clavien–Dindo grade I to V complication rates of mini-PCNL were 2.7–20.8%, 1.4–17.3%, 0–10.3%, 0–0.05% and 0–0.02%, respectively [20]. The results of the current study were within the range and may prove the safety of our technique.

In addition to precise transpapillary renal puncture by ultrasound guidance, the miniaturization of the PCN tract is also associated with less renal trauma and lower bleeding risk and will lead to lower pain scale scores and fewer hemorrhagic complications [9,21]. In the present study, the mean decrease in hemoglobin is 1.04 g/dL. In addition, only two patients experienced bladder blood clot retention and underwent further cystoscopic blood clot evacuation. No patient needed a blood transfusion or radiological intervention for hemorrhage. Contemporary reports of mini-PCNL also showed a very low incidence of blood transfusion (<2%) [20]. Moreover, only 20% of the patients needed postoperative intravenous analgesics. These results indicated the minimal invasiveness of the procedure.

The incidence and severity of postoperative infection were low and acceptable in the present series. It is well known that mini-PCNL with a smaller Amplatz-type renal sheath wall causes higher intrarenal pressure, which leads to pyelovenous backflow [22] and has been identified as a risk factor for sepsis after PCNL [23]. However, the horizontal or downward axis of the Amplatz-type renal sheath in the GMSV position and low irrigation pressure by gravity rather than by irrigation pump decreases the intrarenal pressure significantly and helps to avoid postoperative infection [10]. In addition, the longer operative time is another risk factor for postoperative sepsis after PCNL [23]. However, in the GMSV position, the operative time was reduced not only by a single position throughout the whole procedure but also enhancement of the vacuum cleaner effect associated with the Amplatz-type renal sheath axis. Given the lower intrarenal pressure and shorter operative time in the present study, although 44 patients (29.3%) had positive preoperative urine cultures, only 15 patients (10%) experienced postoperative fever >38 °C, which was transient in most patients. Only two patients (1.3%) developed urosepsis, which was controlled by antibiotics administration. No patients developed septic shock. In the latest meta-analysis, the pooled incidence of fever after mini-PCNL is also about 10% [19]. Additionally, postoperative sepsis developed in 0.9–4.7% of patients after PCNL [20]. The results of current study were similar and acceptable.

The present study has several limitations. First, it was a retrospective, single-center study with the inherent limitations of these design factors. Moreover, it lacked a control group for comparison. The stone-free status was measured by KUB but not by computed tomography, which may lead to the under-detection of residual stone fragments. However, all surgeries were performed by the same urologist (Dr. Yi Yang Liu), which eliminates inter-surgeon bias. To the best of our knowledge, only a few studies have investigated PCNL in combination with the three novel techniques. Therefore, this study is a pioneer in exploring the combined PCNL techniques. Further prospective, multi-institutional comparative studies are still needed to confirm the safety and efficacy of this novel procedure compared to the conventional PCNL. Moreover, this combined technique may be suitable for some special situations, such as urolithiasis in solitary kidneys or transplant kidneys, to avoid severe intraoperative complications [24].

5. Conclusions

In this study, we found that ultrasound guidance, GMSV position and mini-PCNL are mutually complementary. Additionally, balloon dilation of the PCN tract and retrograde semi-rigid ureteroscopic assistance is helpful for renal access creation when performing ultrasound-guided PCNL under the GMSV position. Moreover, low-pressure gravity irrigation under the GMSV position ensures low intrarenal pressure and intraoperative safety. In conclusion, totally X-ray-free ultrasound-guided mini-PCNL in the GMSV position is feasible, safe and effective for patients with renal or upper ureteral stones, indicating the synergistic effects of the three novel techniques.

Author Contributions: Study conception and design: Y.-T.C.; provision of study patients: H.-L.L., Y.-C.S., C.-H.C. and Y.-C.C.; data acquisition: H.-L.L., Y.-C.S., C.-H.C. and Y.-C.C.; data analysis: K.-W.H.; data interpretation: Y.-Y.L. and H.-J.W.; manuscript writing: Y.-Y.L.; manuscript revision: H.-J.W. All authors have read and agreed to the published version of the manuscript.

Funding: This research received no external funding.

Institutional Review Board Statement: The study was conducted in accordance with the Declaration of Helsinki and approved by the Institutional Review Board of Kaohsiung Chang Gung Memorial Hospital (No. 202201106B0, approved on 28 July 2022).

Informed Consent Statement: Due to the retrospective review design of this study, the IRB waived informed consent of the included patients.

Data Availability Statement: The datasets generated during the current study are available from the corresponding author upon reasonable request.

Acknowledgments: We thank all the patients and staff at the Department of Urology of the Kaohsiung Chang Gung Memorial Hospital for their valuable support of this study.

Conflicts of Interest: The authors declare no conflict of interest.

References

1. Fernstrom, I.; Johansson, B. Percutaneous pyelolithotomy. A new extraction technique. *Scand. J. Urol. Nephrol.* **1976**, *10*, 257–259. [CrossRef] [PubMed]
2. Zeng, G.; Zhong, W.; Pearle, M.; Choong, S.; Chew, B.; Skolarikos, A.; Liatsikos, E.; Pal, S.K.; Lahme, S.; Durutovic, O.; et al. European Association of Urology Section of Urolithiasis and International Alliance of Urolithiasis Joint Consensus on Percutaneous Nephrolithotomy. *Eur. Urol. Focus* **2022**, *8*, 588–597. [CrossRef] [PubMed]
3. Ruhayel, Y.; Tepeler, A.; Dabestani, S.; MacLennan, S.; Petrik, A.; Sarica, K.; Seitz, C.; Skolarikos, A.; Straub, M.; Turk, C.; et al. Tract Sizes in Miniaturized Percutaneous Nephrolithotomy: A Systematic Review from the European Association of Urology Urolithiasis Guidelines Panel. *Eur. Urol.* **2017**, *72*, 220–235. [CrossRef] [PubMed]
4. Desai, M.; Ridhorkar, V.; Patel, S.; Bapat, S.; Desai, M. Pediatric percutaneous nephrolithotomy: Assessing impact of technical innovations on safety and efficacy. *J. Endourol.* **1999**, *13*, 359–364. [CrossRef]
5. Lahme, S.; Bichler, K.H.; Strohmaier, W.L.; Gotz, T. Minimally invasive PCNL in patients with renal pelvic and calyceal stones. *Eur. Urol.* **2001**, *40*, 619–624. [CrossRef]
6. Zeng, G.; Cai, C.; Duan, X.; Xu, X.; Mao, H.; Li, X.; Nie, Y.; Xie, J.; Li, J.; Lu, J.; et al. Mini Percutaneous Nephrolithotomy Is a Noninferior Modality to Standard Percutaneous Nephrolithotomy for the Management of 20–40 mm Renal Calculi: A Multicenter Randomized Controlled Trial. *Eur. Urol.* **2021**, *79*, 114–121. [CrossRef]
7. Ibarluzea, G.; Scoffone, C.M.; Cracco, C.M.; Poggio, M.; Porpiglia, F.; Terrone, C.; Astobieta, A.; Camargo, I.; Gamarra, M.; Tempia, A.; et al. Supine Valdivia and modified lithotomy position for simultaneous anterograde and retrograde endourological access. *BJU Int.* **2007**, *100*, 233–236. [CrossRef]
8. Beiko, D.; Razvi, H.; Bhojani, N.; Bjazevic, J.; Bayne, D.B.; Tzou, D.T.; Stoller, M.L.; Chi, T. Techniques–Ultrasound-guided percutaneous nephrolithotomy: How we do it. *Can. Urol. Assoc. J.* **2020**, *14*, E104–E110. [CrossRef]
9. Zhu, W.; Liu, Y.; Liu, L.; Lei, M.; Yuan, J.; Wan, S.P.; Zeng, G. Minimally invasive versus standard percutaneous nephrolithotomy: A meta-analysis. *Urolithiasis* **2015**, *43*, 563–570. [CrossRef]

10. Proietti, S.; Rodriguez-Socarras, M.E.; Eisner, B.; De Coninck, V.; Sofer, M.; Saitta, G.; Rodriguez-Monsalve, M.; D'Orta, C.; Bellinzoni, P.; Gaboardi, F.; et al. Supine percutaneous nephrolithotomy: Tips and tricks. *Transl. Androl. Urol.* **2019**, *8*, S381–S388. [CrossRef]
11. Khazaali, M.; Khazaeli, D.; Moombeini, H.; Jafari-Samim, J. Supine Ultrasound-guided Percutaneous Nephrolithotomy with Retrograde Semi-rigid Ureteroscopic guidwire retrieval: Description of an Evolved Technique. *Urol. J.* **2017**, *14*, 5038–5042. [CrossRef] [PubMed]
12. Li, J.; Gao, L.; Li, Q.; Zhang, Y.; Jiang, Q. Supine versus prone position for percutaneous nephrolithotripsy: A meta-analysis of randomized controlled trials. *Int. J. Surg.* **2019**, *66*, 62–71. [CrossRef] [PubMed]
13. Khadgi, S.; El-Nahas, A.R.; Darrad, M.; Al-Terki, A. Safety and efficacy of a single middle calyx access (MCA) in mini-PCNL. *Urolithiasis* **2020**, *48*, 541–546. [CrossRef] [PubMed]
14. Okhunov, Z.; Friedlander, J.I.; George, A.K.; Duty, B.D.; Moreira, D.M.; Srinivasan, A.K.; Hillelsohn, J.; Smith, A.D.; Okeke, Z. STONE nephrolithometry: Novel surgical classification system for kidney calculi. *Urology* **2013**, *81*, 1154–1159. [CrossRef] [PubMed]
15. Wang, S.; Zhang, Y.; Zhang, X.; Tang, Y.; Xiao, B.; Hu, W.; Chen, S.; Li, J. Tract dilation monitored by ultrasound in percutaneous nephrolithotomy: Feasible and safe. *World J. Urol.* **2020**, *38*, 1569–1576. [CrossRef]
16. Nicklas, A.P.; Schilling, D.; Bader, M.J.; Herrmann, T.R.; Nagele, U.; Training and Research in Urological Surgery and Technology (T.R.U.S.T.)-Group. The vacuum cleaner effect in minimally invasive percutaneous nephrolitholapaxy. *World J. Urol.* **2015**, *33*, 1847–1853. [CrossRef]
17. Zhong, W.; Zeng, G.; Wu, K.; Li, X.; Chen, W.; Yang, H. Does a smaller tract in percutaneous nephrolithotomy contribute to high renal pelvic pressure and postoperative fever? *J. Endourol.* **2008**, *22*, 2147–2151. [CrossRef]
18. DiBianco, J.M.; Ghani, K.R. Precision Stone Surgery: Current Status of Miniaturized Percutaneous Nephrolithotomy. *Curr. Urol. Rep.* **2021**, *22*, 24. [CrossRef]
19. Wan, C.; Wang, D.; Xiang, J.; Yang, B.; Xu, J.; Zhou, G.; Zhou, Y.; Zhao, Y.; Zhong, J.; Liu, J. Comparison of postoperative outcomes of mini percutaneous nephrolithotomy and standard percutaneous nephrolithotomy: A meta-analysis. *Urolithiasis* **2022**, *50*, 523–533. [CrossRef]
20. Singh, H.; Jha, A.K.; Thummar, H.G. Complications in Mini PCNL. In *Minimally Invasive Percutaneous Nephrolithotomy*; Agrawal, M.S., Mishra, D.K., Somani, B., Eds.; Springer: Singapore, 2022; pp. 305–322.
21. Yamaguchi, A.; Skolarikos, A.; Buchholz, N.P.; Chomon, G.B.; Grasso, M.; Saba, P.; Nakada, S.; de la Rosette, J.; Clinical Research Office of the Endourological Society Percutaneous Nephrolithotomy Study Group. Operating times and bleeding complications in percutaneous nephrolithotomy: A comparison of tract dilation methods in 5537 patients in the Clinical Research Office of the Endourological Society Percutaneous Nephrolithotomy Global Study. *J. Endourol.* **2011**, *25*, 933–939. [CrossRef]
22. Boccafoschi, C.; Lugnani, F. Intra-renal reflux. *Urol. Res.* **1985**, *13*, 253–258. [CrossRef] [PubMed]
23. Kreydin, E.I.; Eisner, B.H. Risk factors for sepsis after percutaneous renal stone surgery. *Nat. Rev. Urol.* **2013**, *10*, 598–605. [CrossRef] [PubMed]
24. Sarier, M.; Duman, I.; Yuksel, Y.; Tekin, S.; Demir, M.; Arslan, F.; Ergun, O.; Kosar, A.; Yavuz, A.H. Results of minimally invasive surgical treatment of allograft lithiasis in live-donor renal transplant recipients: A single-center experience of 3758 renal transplantations. *Urolithiasis* **2019**, *47*, 273–278. [CrossRef] [PubMed]

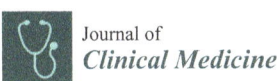

Journal of Clinical Medicine

Article

Variation in Tap Water Mineral Content in the United Kingdom: Is It Relevant for Kidney Stone Disease?

Kirolos G. F. T. Michael [1] and Bhaskar K. Somani [2,*]

[1] Northern Care Alliance NHS Foundation Trust, Salford M6 8HD, UK
[2] Department of Urology, University Hospital Southampton, Southampton SO16 6YD, UK
* Correspondence: bhaskarsomani@yahoo.com; Tel.: +44-23-8120-6873

Abstract: Introduction: The dissolved mineral content of drinking water can modify a number of excreted urinary parameters, with potential implications for kidney stone disease (KSD). The aim of this study is to investigate the variation in the mineral content of tap drinking water in the United Kingdom and discuss its implications for KSD. Methods: The mineral composition of tap water from cities across the United Kingdom was ascertained from publicly available water quality reports issued by local water supply companies using civic centre postcodes during 2021. Water variables, reported as 12-monthly average values, included total water hardness and concentrations of calcium, magnesium, sodium and sulphate. An unpaired t-test was undertaken to assess for regional differences in water composition across the United Kingdom. Results: Water composition data were available for 66 out of 76 cities in the United Kingdom: 45 in England, 8 in Scotland, 7 in Wales and 6 in Northern Ireland. The median water hardness in the United Kingdom was 120.59 mg/L $CaCO_3$ equivalent (range 16.02–331.50), while the median concentrations of calcium, magnesium, sodium and sulphate were 30.46 mg/L (range 5.35–128.0), 3.62 mg/L (range 0.59–31.80), 14.72 mg/L (range 2.98–57.80) and 25.36 mg/L (range 2.86–112.43), respectively. Tap water in England was markedly harder than in Scotland (192.90 mg/L vs. 32.87 mg/L as $CaCO_3$ equivalent; $p < 0.001$), which overall had the softest tap water with the lowest mineral content in the United Kingdom. Within England, the North West had the softest tap water, while the South East had the hardest water (70.00 mg/L vs. 285.75 mg/L as $CaCO_3$ equivalent). Conclusions: Tap water mineral content varies significantly across the United Kingdom. Depending on where one lives, drinking 2–3 L of tap water can contribute over one-third of recommended daily calcium and magnesium requirements, with possible implications for KSD incidence and recurrence.

Keywords: urolithiasis; kidney calculi; tap water; mineral composition; kidney stones

Citation: Michael, K.G.F.T.; Somani, B.K. Variation in Tap Water Mineral Content in the United Kingdom: Is It Relevant for Kidney Stone Disease? *J. Clin. Med.* **2022**, *11*, 5118. https://doi.org/10.3390/jcm11175118

Academic Editors: Francisco Guillen-Grima and Ersilia Lucenteforte

Received: 2 August 2022
Accepted: 28 August 2022
Published: 30 August 2022

Publisher's Note: MDPI stays neutral with regard to jurisdictional claims in published maps and institutional affiliations.

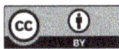

Copyright: © 2022 by the authors. Licensee MDPI, Basel, Switzerland. This article is an open access article distributed under the terms and conditions of the Creative Commons Attribution (CC BY) license (https://creativecommons.org/licenses/by/4.0/).

1. Introduction

The aetiology of kidney stone disease (KSD) is complex and is the product of the intricate interplay between dietary, lifestyle, environmental and genetic factors which predispose individuals to disease [1]. In the United Kingdom, the prevalence of KSD is rising, with an estimated 1 in 7 individuals requiring intervention during their lifetime, posing a substantial burden to health services [2,3]. There is therefore great impetus for investigating factors implicated in KSD, which may lead to more specific preventative strategies.

At present, the mainstay of KSD prevention is to advise patients to increase their daily fluid intake [4,5]. Nevertheless, whether or not the type of fluid matters is still debatable. Amongst studies conducted to investigate whether any type of water is superior for patients with KSD, there is a weak consensus that mineral-rich water may result in favourable changes to urine composition, which may reduce the risk of calcium stone formation [6]. For this reason, a number of studies have sought to compare the mineral composition of drinking water, whether bottled or supplied through taps, to further study the association between water composition and KSD [7–9].

Drinking water supplied through taps is derived from different sources depending on the region, leading to variations in its dissolved mineral content. [10] The "hardness" of tap water reflects the quantity of dissolved metal ions, principally calcium and magnesium [11]. Given the recognised implications of drinking water on human health, most countries monitor and tightly regulate tap water quality and composition, though recommended ranges and maximum values are largely not based on research [12]. In the United Kingdom, governmental studies have revealed that up to 97% of adults drink tap water, with the average adult consuming 1.3 L of tap water per day, accounting for nearly two-thirds of daily fluid consumption in England and Wales [13]. Given these findings, the aim of this study is to investigate the variation in tap water composition across the United Kingdom and describe potential implications for KSD.

2. Materials and Methods

The mineral composition of tap water during 2021 across all officially designated cities in the United Kingdom was investigated from online, publicly available water quality reports obtained from the local water supply company using the postcode of the city hall or civic centre, as a representative of the area. Where reports were not available online, water supply companies were contacted directly to request these. Cities that did not have water quality reports covering 2021 were excluded. Water variables collected included total water hardness, in addition to the concentrations of calcium, magnesium, sodium and sulphate where available. Values obtained represent an average value over a 12-month period for a given area. Potassium and bicarbonate concentrations were not included due to insufficient data across the regions to enable comparison.

To determine whether tap water mineral composition varies significantly between regions of the United Kingdom, a pairwise comparison of mean water variables was undertaken between constituent countries in the United Kingdom. Statistical analysis was undertaken using SPSS Statistics for Windows, version 25 (IBM Corp., Armonk, NY, USA), and statistical significance was determined at the ≤ 0.05 level.

3. Results

3.1. Comparison of Water Composition across Constituent Countries in the United Kingdom

In total, 66 out of 76 cities in the United Kingdom were included in this study: 45 in England, 8 in Scotland, 7 in Wales and 6 in Northern Ireland. Tap water was supplied to these by 17 different water supply companies across the United Kingdom.

The median water hardness in the United Kingdom was 120.59 mg/L $CaCO_3$ equivalent (range: 16.02–331.50). The median concentrations of calcium, magnesium, sodium and sulphate were 30.46 mg/L (range: 5.35–128.0), 3.62 mg/L (range: 0.59–31.80), 14.72 mg/L (range: 2.98–57.80) and 25.36 mg/L (range: 2.86–112.43), respectively.

A comparison of the median values and ranges of water composition variables of interest between countries in the United Kingdom is presented in Table 1 and Figure 1. Compared to Scotland, which had the lowest mineral content, tap water in England was significantly harder (192.90 mg/L vs. 32.87 mg/L as $CaCO_3$ equivalent) and had a higher concentration of calcium (77.56 mg/L vs. 10.69 mg/L), magnesium (4.65 mg/L vs. 1.59 mg/L), sodium (17.90 mg/L vs. 6.39 mg/L) and sulphate (37.00 mg/L vs. 9.07 mg/L) when comparing median values. A pairwise comparison of mean water variables revealed statistically significant differences between water composition values across the United Kingdom (Table 2).

Table 1. Comparison of water composition by country in the United Kingdom.

Country	Median Total Hardness/mg/L [Range]	Median Calcium Concentration/mg/L [Range]	Median Magnesium Concentration/mg/L [Range]	Median Sodium Concentration/mg/L [Range]	Median Sulphate Concentration/mg/L [Range]
England	192.90 [19.00–331.50]	77.56 [6.73–128.00]	4.65 [1.30–31.80]	17.90 [2.98–57.80]	37.00 [7.95–112.43]
Scotland	32.87 [16.02–52.38]	10.69 [5.35–17.73]	1.59 [0.65–2.02]	6.39 [3.93–8.23]	9.07 [2.86–18.38]
Wales	68.93 [26.15–124.29]	26.83 [8.98–36.93]	3.88 [0.59–7.14]	10.93 [5.99–22.70]	6.74 [6.74–37.30]
Northern Ireland	100.95 [24.40–141.50]	31.50 [8.60–56.60]	5.35 [0.70–8.90]	N.D.	N.D.
Total	120.59 [16.02–331.50]	30.46 [5.35–128.00]	3.62 [0.59–31.80]	14.72 [2.98–57.80]	25.36 [2.86–112.43]

N.D. denotes no data available.

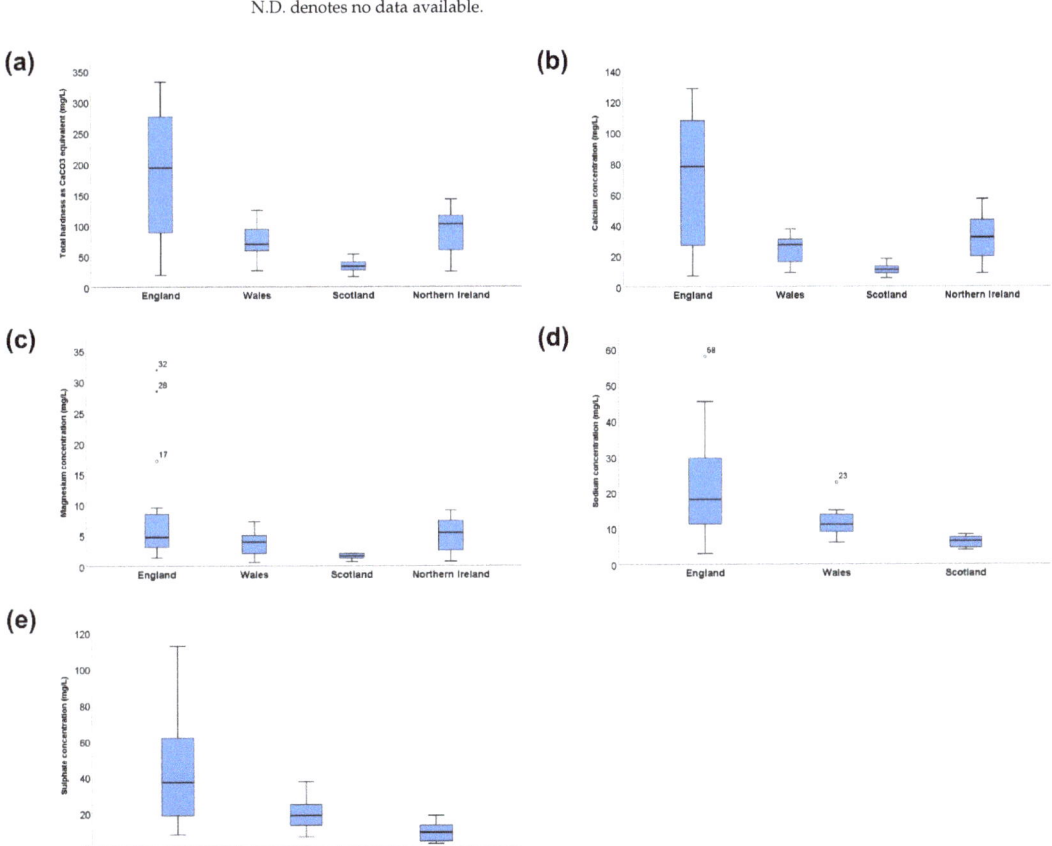

Figure 1. Distribution of the mineral composition of tap water across the United Kingdom. Mineral composition of tap water by country (mg/L). (**a**) Total water hardness as CaCO3 equivalent (**b**) Calcium concentration (**c**) Magnesium concentration (**d**) Sodium concentration (**e**) Sulphate concentration. ○ Outlier (value > 1.5 IQR); ★ Extreme outlier (value > 3 IQR). N.D. denotes no data available.

Table 2. Pairwise t-test significance values for differences in mean water variables by country in the United Kingdom.

Total Water Hardness				
	England	*Wales*	*Scotland*	*Northern Ireland*
England		0.001	<0.001	0.009
Wales	0.001		0.005	0.460
Scotland	<0.001	0.005		0.003
Northern Ireland	0.009	0.460	0.003	
Calcium				
	England	*Wales*	*Scotland*	*Northern Ireland*
England		0.016	0.001	0.044
Wales	0.016		0.006	0.381
Scotland	0.001	0.006		0.005
Northern Ireland	0.044	0.381	0.005	
Magnesium				
	England	*Wales*	*Scotland*	*Northern Ireland*
England		0.283	0.048	0.044
Wales	0.283		0.020	0.443
Scotland	0.048	0.020		0.010
Northern Ireland	0.492	0.443	0.010	
Sodium				
	England	*Wales*	*Scotland*	*Northern Ireland*
England		0.057	0.001	N.D.
Wales	0.057		0.011	N.D.
Scotland	0.001	0.011		N.D.
Northern Ireland	N.D.	N.D.	N.D.	
Sulphate				
	England	*Wales*	*Scotland*	*Northern Ireland*
England		0.041	0.001	N.D.
Wales	0.041		0.033	N.D.
Scotland	0.001	0.033		N.D.
Northern Ireland	N.D.	N.D.	N.D.	

N.D. denotes no data available; *p* values in bold are statistically significant at the 0.05 level.

3.2. Regional Variation in Tap Water Composition across England

Given the wide range of water variables in England, a comparison of tap water composition across the different regions of England was undertaken. Cities in eight out of the nine regions in England had freely available water quality reports from 2021, with no cities in the Yorkshire and the Humber region reporting water composition beyond 2020 at the time of the investigation. The differences in water composition across the eight regions are presented in Table 3 and Figure 2. Even within England, there was a four-fold difference between the region with the hardest tap water (South East) and the region with the softest water (North West). Similarly, there was approximately a six-fold difference between the region with the highest calcium concentration (East) and the North West, as well as a near the 13-fold difference between the region with the highest magnesium concentration (East Midlands) and the North West.

Table 3. Comparison of water composition by region in England.

Region	Median Total Hardness/mg/L [Range]	Median Calcium Concentration/mg/L [Range]	Median Magnesium Concentration/mg/L [Range]	Median Sodium Concentration/mg/L [Range]	Median Sulfate Concentration/mg/L [Range]
East	269.00 [182.28–331.50]	104.90 [78.10–128.00]	8.74 [2.07–17.10]	28.40 [10.10–57.80]	59.79 [20.00–111.00]
East Midlands	165.90 [148.25–192.80]	59.30 [59.30–59.30]	31.80 [31.80–31.80]	29.80 [25.00–37.00]	64.00 [50.00–87.60]
London	272.00 [271.00–273.00]	N.D.	4.30 [4.20–4.30]	28.60 [27.60–29.60]	47.35 [46.40–48.30]
North East	116.88 [50.03–277.43]	38.05 [16.67–77.01]	5.29 [2.03–28.33]	17.33 [7.98–43.35]	61.35 [29.87–112.43]
North West	70.00 [19.00–109.00]	17.90 [6.73–33.60]	2.49 [1.30–6.13]	14.50 [2.98–19.00]	26.10 [7.95–42.80]
South East	285.75 [257.00–302.00]	104.72 [97.00–112.43]	4.80 [3.00–7.98]	14.93 [9.03–42.90]	20.29 [12.91–109.00]
South West	185.30 [39.98–33–.38]	97.085 [62.00–119.66]	6.30 [4.50–8.10]	10.60 [8.20–45.30]	14.60 [9.00–86.00]
West Midlands	156.25 [51.10–212.40]	27.58 [27.58–27.58]	3.10 [3.10–3.10]	16.60 [11.10–35.90]	34.65 [21.00–64.00]
Total	192.80 [19.00–331.50]	77.56 [6.73–128.00]	4.65 [1.30–31.80]	17.90 [2.98–57.80]	37.00 [7.95–112.43]

N.D. denotes no data available.

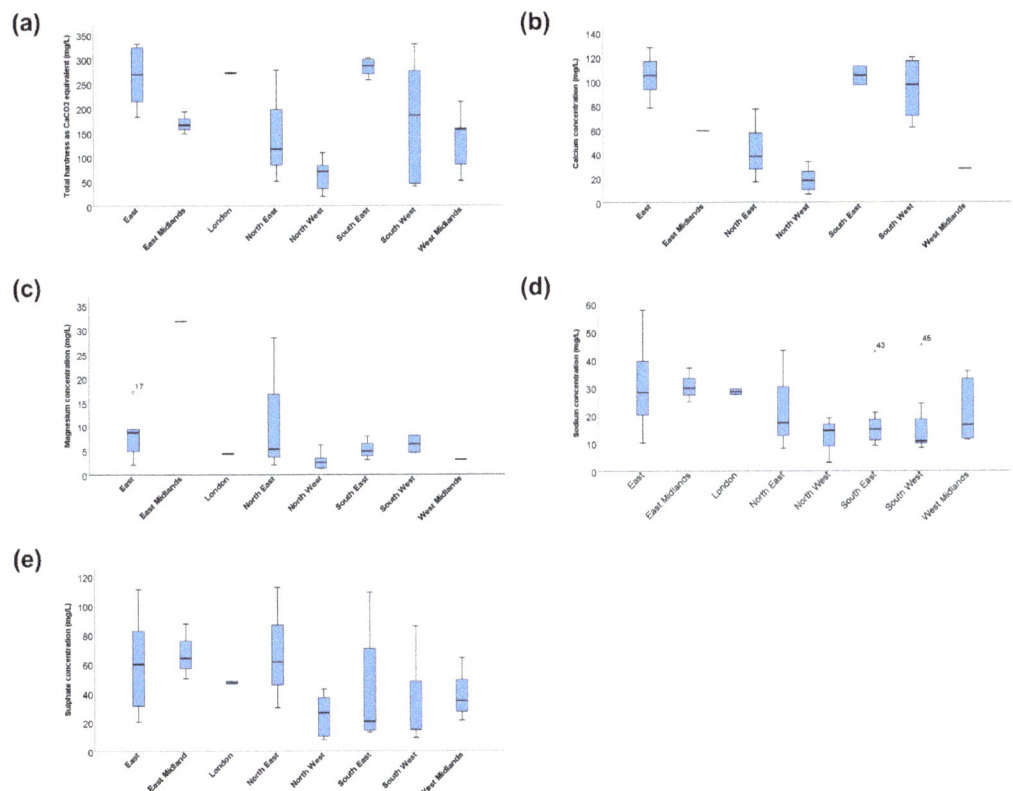

Figure 2. Distribution of the mineral composition of tap water across England Mineral composition of tap water by region (mg/L). (**a**) Total water hardness as CaCO3 equivalent (**b**) Calcium concentration (**c**) Magnesium concentration (**d**) Sodium concentration (**e**) Sulphate concentration. ○ Outlier (value > 1.5 IQR); ★ Extreme outlier (value > 3 IQR).

3.3. Comparison of Bottled Water and Tap Water

Tap water mineral content in the United Kingdom was compared to that of commonly available bottled water brands comprising 11 brands of still water and 6 of sparkling water, as previously described by Stoots et al. (Table 4) [8]. Compared to bottled still and sparkling water from popular brands in the United Kingdom, tap water had a lower median calcium and magnesium concentration but a greater range in these values overall. By contrast, tap water had a higher sodium and sulphate content compared to bottled water.

Table 4. Comparison of bottled and tap water in the United Kingdom.

	Median Calcium Concentration/mg/L [Range]	Median Magnesium Concentration/mg/L [Range]	Median Sodium Concentration/mg/L [Range]	Median Sulphate Concentration/mg/L [Range]
Bottled still [8]	55.00 [12.00–59.00]	10.05 [3.50–19.00]	11.90 [7.03–12.00]	12.00 [9.00–14.00]
Bottled sparkling [8]	56.00 [55.00–104.00]	18.00 [10.00–19.00]	11.50 [7.47–24.00]	13.00 [9.00–28.00]
Tap water	30.46 [5.35–128.00]	3.62 [0.59–31.80]	14.72 [2.98–57.8]	25.36 [2.86–112.43]

4. Discussion

4.1. Findings from Our Study

Our study described the variation in the mineral composition of drinking water supplied through taps across the United Kingdom. We found significant regional variation in tap water hardness and calcium, magnesium, sodium and sulphate concentrations of tap water. Notably, we report a 24-fold and 54-fold difference between the maximum and minimum tap water calcium and magnesium concentrations across regions of the United Kingdom. Interestingly, whilst bottled water, on average, had higher concentrations of most minerals of interest, the ranges of these values for tap water were larger. As far as the authors are aware, this study is the first to compare tap water mineral content across the different cities and regions of the United Kingdom.

4.2. Mineral Content and Pathogenesis of KSD

A number of minerals present in drinking water likely play a role in the pathogenesis of KSD, particularly calcium, magnesium and sodium. At present, the literature is in agreement that moderate calcium intake is protective against KSD, though supplemental calcium may not be beneficial and could, on the contrary, increase the risk of calcium nephrolithiasis, especially if taken separately from meals [14]. Likewise, the role of magnesium in protecting against KSD is widely recognised, while sulphate may be protective against calcium nephrolithiasis by reducing ionised urinary calcium and supersaturation of calcium salts [6,15–17]. Conversely, sodium in the form of salt (sodium chloride) is a well-established risk factor for calcium nephrolithiasis, and it is a routine clinical practice to counsel patients at risk of KSD to reduce their salt intake [18].

4.3. Comparison with Previous Studies

Several studies investigating tap water mineral variation have been undertaken, with comparable findings. In the Flanders region of Belgium, tap water mineral content was found to vary significantly, with a 10-fold and 12-fold difference between the highest and lowest calcium and magnesium concentrations with similar maximum values reported compared to the United Kingdom [9]. Similarly, in Australia, tap water calcium was found to vary regionally by a factor of 15.6, while magnesium varied by a factor of 10.7, though unlike in Flanders, the mineral content of tap water overall was significantly lower compared to the United Kingdom, with the maximum calcium and magnesium concentrations being approximately 6-times and 3-times lower [19]. In North America, one study found a 42-fold difference in tap water calcium concentration, while there was a 48-fold difference in magnesium concentration between regions with the highest and lowest concentrations [20]. It should be noted that these comparisons are, in most cases,

4.4. Implications for Clinical Practice

For adults living in the United Kingdom, the recommended daily intake for calcium is 700 mg/d, while for magnesium, it is 300 mg/d (males) or 270 mg (females); for sodium, it is 2400 mg/d [21]. Our study found that depending on where one lives, drinking 2 L of tap water can contribute 1.5–36.6% of recommended daily calcium intake and 0.4–23.6% of daily magnesium intake, making tap water a significant but often overlooked source of these minerals. By contrast, tap water contributes 0.2–4.7% of daily sodium intake, which is relatively insignificant compared to other dietary sources. Furthermore, the proportion of calcium and magnesium derived from tap water is likely to be even higher for KSD patients, who will often be advised to drink up to 3 L of fluid per day. The British Association of Urological Surgeons (BAUS) includes advice on calcium intake in its "dietary advice for stone formers" patient information leaflet, highlighting that daily intake of up to 1,000 mg of calcium is safe whilst also detailing the calcium content of a number of dairy products for reference [22]. Our finding that tap water in the United Kingdom can be a significant contributor to daily calcium intake raises an interesting question: should clinicians routinely advise KSD patients to be mindful of the mineral content of their tap water? Similarly, should such advice be included on patient information leaflets?

Having recognised that significant variations in the mineral content of tap water exist regionally and globally and that tap water can be a significant contributor to daily calcium and magnesium intake, the question then becomes whether these regional variations are of clinical significance when it comes to KSD incidence and recurrence. A number of interventional studies have demonstrated that consumption of drinking water with different mineral compositions can result in changes to excreted urinary calcium, magnesium and citrate levels as well as urinary pH, with a weak consensus in the literature favouring hard, mineral-rich water for patients at risk of KSD [6]. When compared to tap water in our study, the mineral content of different types of water included in these study protocols was, for the most part, within the ranges of total hardness, calcium and magnesium levels in tap water in the United Kingdom, although the maximum calcium concentrations in some of the studies were significantly higher, being derived from bottled mineral water [23–25]. It can therefore be hypothesised that variation in the mineral content of tap water in the United Kingdom may translate into variations in excreted urinary parameters of key promoting and inhibitory lithogenic factors. This is supported by a large North American study which found that 24-h urine calcium, magnesium and citrate increased with tap water hardness [26]. Nevertheless, the same study did not find large differences in the number of lifetime KSD episodes between those living in regions with soft versus hard water, though dietary, metabolic and other environmental risk factors for urolithiasis were not controlled for. Moreover, in Iran, a weak inverse correlation was demonstrated between tap water magnesium concentration and KSD incidence, further raising the possibility that tap water variations may be implicated in KSD incidence [27].

4.5. Limitations and Future Direction

A number of limitations are present in our study. Since water composition data were derived from 19 different water supply companies providing for the 66 cities included in our study, there was a degree of heterogeneity in how tap water quality and composition were reported between companies. Though all values were reported as a 12-monthly average, with most companies reporting mean values, for others, it was not clear what kind of average was reported. Furthermore, a number of water supply companies did not report all variables of interest in this study, though every company reported total water hardness, and the vast majority reported calcium and magnesium levels. Few reports included pH, bicarbonate and potassium levels and hence were not included in our study since meaningful comparisons between regions could not be undertaken. While our study described variations in tap water mineral composition, it did not relate this to KSD incidence or recurrence. Finally, we considered the mineral content of tap water in light of KSD; however, there are a number of other conditions, including mineral bone disease, that may be impacted by drinking water mineral composition, which should not be neglected when advising patients on the optimal type of water [28]. To further investigate the association between tap water and KSD, future studies should explore whether variation in tap water mineral content correlates with KSD incidence. Additionally, it would be interesting to determine whether there are significant regional variations in urinary calculus composition and, if so, whether these correlate with any tap water variable since different types of calculi may be impacted in different ways by different types of water. In the future, it would also be interesting to perform additional epidemiological studies, in particular ecological studies related to water composition and incidence of KSD.

5. Conclusions

The mineral content of tap water varies significantly between different regions in the United Kingdom. Depending on where one lives, drinking 2–3 L of tap water per day can contribute over one-third of recommended daily calcium and magnesium intake, making tap water a significant but often overlooked source of these minerals. Whilst the exact relationship between drinking water mineral content and KSD incidence and recurrence has yet to be fully elucidated, clinicians should be mindful that in some regions, tap water can be a significant source of important minerals such as calcium, especially when counselling patients already on supplementation for other medical conditions. Future studies should focus on tailoring preventative strategies related to fluid consumption to the type of drinking water available to patients, 24-h urine chemistries and calculus composition to deliver more effective, personalised preventative strategies for patients at risk of recurrence.

Author Contributions: K.G.F.T.M.: Methodology, investigation, visualisation, writing—original draft preparation; B.K.S.: conceptualisation, supervision, writing—review and editing. All authors have read and agreed to the published version of the manuscript.

Funding: No funds: grants or other support was received for conducting this study.

Institutional Review Board Statement: This study does not describe research on patients or human subjects and hence did not require ethical approval.

Informed Consent Statement: Informed consent was not required, as it is a review article.

Data Availability Statement: Data generated and analysed are included in this study. Further enquiries can be directed to the corresponding author regarding acquisition of water quality reports used in this investigation.

Conflicts of Interest: The authors have no conflict of interest, financial or otherwise, to declare.

References

1. Dawson, C.H.; Tomson, C.R. Kidney stone disease: Pathophysiology, investigation and medical treatment. *Clin. Med.* **2012**, *12*, 467–471. [CrossRef] [PubMed]
2. Rukin, N.J.; Siddiqui, Z.A.; Chedgy, E.C.; Somani, B.K. Trends in Upper Tract Stone Disease in England: Evidence from the Hospital Episodes Statistics Database. *Urol. Int.* **2017**, *98*, 391–396. [CrossRef] [PubMed]
3. Geraghty, R.M.; Cook, P.; Walker, V.; Somani, B.K. Evaluation of the economic burden of kidney stone disease in the UK: A retrospective cohort study with a mean follow-up of 19 years. *Br. J. Urol. Int.* **2020**, *125*, 586–594. [CrossRef]
4. Bao, Y.; Tu, X.; Wei, Q. Water for preventing urinary stones. *Cochrane Database Syst. Rev.* **2020**, CD004292. [CrossRef]
5. Anonymous. NICE Guideline—Renal and ureteric stones: Assessment and management. *Br. J. Urol. Int.* **2019**, *123*, 220–232. [CrossRef]
6. Sulaiman, S.K.; Enakshee, J.; Traxer, O.; Somani, B.K. Which Type of Water Is Recommended for Patients with Stone Disease (Hard or Soft Water, Tap or Bottled Water): Evidence from a Systematic Review over the Last 3 Decades. *Curr. Urol. Rep.* **2020**, *21*, 6. [CrossRef]

7. Stoots, S.J.; Geraghty, R.; Kamphuis, G.M.; Jamnadass, E.; Henderickx, M.M.; Ventimiglia, E.; Traxer, O.; Keller, E.X.; De Coninck, V.; Talso, M.; et al. Variations in the Mineral Content of Bottled "Still" Water Across Europe: Comparison of 182 Brands Across 10 Countries. *J. Endourol.* **2021**, *35*, 206–214. [CrossRef]
8. Stoots, S.; Kamphuis, G.; Geraghty, R.; Vogt, L.; Henderickx, M.; Hameed, B.; Ibrahim, S.; Pietropaolo, A.; Jamnadass, E.; Aljumaiah, S.; et al. Global Variations in the Mineral Content of Bottled Still and Sparkling Water and a Description of the Possible Impact on Nephrological and Urological Diseases. *J. Clin. Med.* **2021**, *10*, 2807. [CrossRef] [PubMed]
9. Henderickx, M.M.E.L.; Stoots, S.J.M.; Baard, J.; Kamphuis, G.M. Could the region you live in prevent or precipitate kidney stone formation due to mineral intake through tap water? An analysis of nine distribution regions in Flanders. *Acta Chir. Belg.* **2022**, 1–8. [CrossRef]
10. World Health Organisation. Hardness in Drinking-Water. 2011. Available online: https://www.who.int/water_sanitation_health/dwq/chemicals/hardness.pdf (accessed on 25 June 2022).
11. McGowan, W. *Water Processing: Residential, Commercial, Light-Industrial*, 3rd ed.; Water Quality Association: Lisle, IL, USA, 2000.
12. Kozisek, F. Regulations for calcium, magnesium or hardness in drinking water in the European Union member states. *Regul. Toxicol. Pharmacol.* **2020**, *112*, 104589. [CrossRef]
13. Anonymous. National Tap Water Consumption Survey for England and Wales. n.d. Available online: https://www.dwi.gov.uk/research/completed-research/consumer/national-tap-water-consumption-survey-for-england-and-wales/ (accessed on 12 July 2021).
14. Sorensen, M.D. Calcium intake and urinary stone disease. *Transl. Androl. Urol.* **2014**, *3*, 235–240. [CrossRef] [PubMed]
15. Riley, J.M.; Kim, H.; Averch, T.D.; Kim, H.J. Effect of Magnesium on Calcium and Oxalate Ion Binding. *J. Endourol.* **2013**, *27*, 1487–1492. [CrossRef] [PubMed]
16. Massey, L. Magnesium therapy for nephrolithiasis. *Magnes. Res.* **2005**, *18*, 123–126. [PubMed]
17. Rodgers, A.; Gauvin, D.; Edeh, S.; Allie-Hamdulay, S.; Jackson, G.; Lieske, J.C. Sulfate but Not Thiosulfate Reduces Calculated and Measured Urinary Ionized Calcium and Supersaturation: Implications for the Treatment of Calcium Renal Stones. *PLoS ONE* **2014**, *9*, e103602. [CrossRef] [PubMed]
18. Ticinesi, A.; Nouvenne, A.; Maalouf, N.M.; Borghi, L.; Meschi, T. Salt and nephrolithiasis. *Nephrol. Dial. Transplant.* **2016**, *31*, 39–45. [CrossRef]
19. Kwok, M.; McGeorge, S.; Roberts, M.; Somani, B.; Rukin, N. Mineral content variations between Australian tap and bottled water in the context of urolithiasis. *BJUI Compass* **2022**, *3*, 377–382. [CrossRef]
20. Azoulay, A.; Garzon, P.; Eisenberg, M.J. Comparison of the mineral content of tap water and bottled waters. *J. Gen. Intern. Med.* **2001**, *16*, 168–175. [CrossRef]
21. Public Health England NST. Government Dietary Recommendations Government Recommendations for Energy and Nutrients for Males and Females Aged 1–18 Years and 19+ Years. 2016. Available online: https://www.gov.uk/government/publications/the-eatwell-guide (accessed on 12 July 2022).
22. The British Association of Urological Surgeons. Dietary Advice for Stone Formers. 2021. Available online: https://www.baus.org.uk/professionals/baus_business/news/208/stone_diet_patient_information_leaflet (accessed on 12 July 2022).
23. Bellizzi, V.; DeNicola, L.; Minutolo, R.; Russo, D.; Cianciaruso, B.; Andreucci, M.; Conte, G.; Andreucci, V. Effects of Water Hardness on Urinary Risk Factors for Kidney Stones in Patients with Idiopathic Nephrolithiasis. *Nephron Exp. Nephrol.* **1999**, *81*, 66–70. [CrossRef]
24. Siener, R.; Jahnen, A.; Hesse, A. Influence of a mineral water rich in calcium, magnesium and bicarbonate on urine composition and the risk of calcium oxalate crystallization. *Eur. J. Clin. Nutr.* **2004**, *58*, 270–276. [CrossRef]
25. Mirzazadeh, M.; Nouran, M.G.; Richards, K.A.; Zare, M. Effects of Drinking Water Quality on Urinary Parameters in Men with and Without Urinary Tract Stones. *Urology* **2012**, *79*, 501–507. [CrossRef]
26. Schwartz, B.F.; Schenkman, N.S.; Bruce, J.E.; Leslie, S.W.; Stoller, M.L. Calcium nephrolithiasis: Effect of water hardness on urinary electrolytes. *Urology* **2002**, *60*, 23–27. [CrossRef]
27. Basiri, A.; Shakhssalim, N.; Khoshdel, A.R.; Pakmanesh, H.; Radfar, M.H. Drinking water composition and incidence of urinary calculus: Introducing a new index. *Iran. J. Kidney Dis.* **2011**, *5*, 15–20. [PubMed]
28. Quattrini, S. Natural mineral waters: Chemical characteristics and health effects. *Clin. Cases Miner. Bone Metab.* **2016**, *13*, 173–180. [CrossRef]

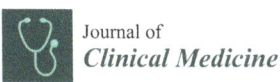

Article

Comparison of the Safety and Efficacy of Laser Versus Pneumatic Intracorporeal Lithotripsy for Treatment of Bladder Stones in Children

Ziad H. Abd [1,*] and Samir A. Muter [2]

1 Department of Surgery, College of Medicine, University of Anbar, Ramadi 31001, Iraq
2 Department of Surgery, College of Medicine, University of Baghdad, Baghdad 10001, Iraq; Samir.muter@yahoo.com
* Correspondence: ziadhabd@uoanbar.edu.iq

Abstract: This study aimed to compare the safety and efficacy of laser lithotripsy and pneumatic lithotripsy, the two most commonly used transurethral lithotripsy methods for treating bladder stones in children in Iraq. Between January 2013 and December 2016, 64 children with bladder stones were included in this prospective randomized study, after ethical committee approval and written consent from the children's parents or caregivers were obtained. Patients were assigned randomly by computer software to two groups treated with either pneumatic cystolithotripsy or laser lithotripsy. A 9 Fr. semirigid ureteroscope was used to pass the lithotripter through and fragment the stone. A catheter of 8–12 Fr. was then introduced and kept in place for 24 h. All children were hospitalized for 24 h, and the catheter was removed the next morning. Outpatient follow-up was maintained for 6–12 months. In terms of operation outcomes and complications, the laser lithotripsy group had a significantly longer duration of operation (74.5 ± 26.6 min vs. 51.5 ± 17.2 min, $p = 0.001$), whereas the number of patients requiring an extended hospital stay was significantly higher in the pneumatic lithotripsy group (48.5% vs. 16.1%, $p = 0.006$). Moreover, pneumatic lithotripsy was associated with a significantly greater risk of having at least one adverse effect (64% greater than that in the laser group). Stone clearance rates did not significantly differ between treatment groups. In conclusion, both pneumatic and laser lithotripters can be used to treat children with bladder stones with high efficacy and safety.

Keywords: laser lithotripsy; pediatric urolithiasis; pneumatic lithotripsy; vesical stone

Citation: Abd, Z.H.; Muter, S.A. Comparison of the Safety and Efficacy of Laser Versus Pneumatic Intracorporeal Lithotripsy for Treatment of Bladder Stones in Children. *J. Clin. Med.* **2022**, *11*, 513. https://doi.org/10.3390/jcm11030513

Academic Editors: Bhaskar K Somani and Kent Doi

Received: 3 January 2022
Accepted: 17 January 2022
Published: 20 January 2022

Publisher's Note: MDPI stays neutral with regard to jurisdictional claims in published maps and institutional affiliations.

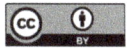

Copyright: © 2022 by the authors. Licensee MDPI, Basel, Switzerland. This article is an open access article distributed under the terms and conditions of the Creative Commons Attribution (CC BY) license (https://creativecommons.org/licenses/by/4.0/).

1. Introduction

Endemic bladder stones in children account for a substantial urologic workload in hospitals in many developing countries despite having nearly disappeared in developed countries as early as 1920 [1]. Iraq and the entire Middle East lies in the Afro-Asian "stone belt", a region with an increased incidence of bladder stones [2]. Compared with those in adults, bladder stones in children are associated with metabolic, nutritional and genetic factors. Dehydration and infection play major roles in bladder stone formation in children [3,4]. Ammonium urate and calcium oxalate stones have been attributed to poor nutrition and low-protein and high-carbohydrate diets [5]. Infants in underdeveloped countries are mainly fed human breast milk and cereals, particularly polished rice, both of which contain low phosphorus content. Low phosphorus diets increase urinary ammonium content [5], thus potentially explaining the high prevalence of bladder stones in developing countries.

Historically, bladder stones were treated with open cystolithotomy, although this procedure is currently rarely needed. Percutaneous cystolithotomy and extracorporeal shock-wave lithotripsy were introduced later during the last century [6]. Although cystolitholapaxy and cystolithotripsy (CL) are the standard treatment modalities for adult bladder stones, a transurethral approach to bladder stones in children was previously not recommended because of a lack of availability of small instruments and the risk of injuring the narrow urethra and causing lifelong urethral stricture disease [7]. Shock-wave treatment of bladder stones in children has been associated with a high re-treatment rate and difficulties in passing the stone fragments [8]. However, after smaller pediatric cystoscopes and pneumatic and laser lithotripters became available, a rapid shift toward the use of less invasive transurethral CL for treating pediatric bladder stones resulted. In 1994, Shokier reported the safe use of a pneumatic lithotripter to fragment bladder stones in children [9]. Subsequently, in 2005, Ramakrishnan et al. used a laser (Ho:YAG) for the same purpose and reported the method to be safe and successful [10]. Since then, many studies have confirmed the safe and efficient use of both modalities in the treatment of pediatric bladder stones. Recently, minimally invasive surgery (MIS) has shown to be safe and effective in removing big bladder stones [11]. The superior advantage of MIS is the possibility of removing bladder stones through the navel, utilizing an endobag, without crushing them [11]. Moreover, robot-assisted laparoscopic surgery has demonstrated efficacy in the treatment of large-volume stones, especially in conditions requiring simultaneous reconstruction [12]. However, robotic surgery in pediatric bladder stones or urolithiasis still needs more evidence to be implemented within the practice [13,14].

Although pneumatic lithotripters have been available in Iraq for many years, laser lithotripters have only recently been introduced and begun to be used by a few urologists. However, other urologists were hesitant to use the laser with concerns related to costs and questionable superiority over pneumatic lithotripters.

We hypothesized that laser CL has equal efficacy and safety compared to pneumatic CL in pediatric bladder stones and that the higher cost of the procedure is outweighed by a lower complication rate and shorter hospital stay.

This study aimed to compare the safety and efficacy of the two transurethral lithotripters most commonly used in the treatment of pediatric bladder stones in Iraq in terms of efficacy and safety. This study has a superior contribution to the field given its prospective design and large sample size compared to previous trials.

2. Materials and Methods

Between January 2013 and December 2016, all children aged 12 years or less and diagnosed with single bladder stones were enrolled in this prospective randomized study after obtaining the ethical committee approval from University of Anbar, College of Medicine with an ethical code of 128EA and written consents from the children's parents or caregivers. All patients belonged to a single ethnic group, Arab.

Exclusion criteria were the presence of active urinary tract infection, multiple bladder stones, urinary tract functional or anatomical abnormality, or previous urinary tract surgical intervention.

After taking a full medical history and performing full clinical examinations on all children, we sent them for laboratory investigations. Laboratory investigations included full blood count, renal function test (electrolytes, urea and creatinine) and urinalysis. Urine culture was ordered only if the urine test showed WBCs > 3 or a UTI was clinically suspected because of the limited availability of culture media in the hospital at the time the study was conducted. Patient imaging was used to make the initial diagnosis and then reviewed by the treating consultant, and additional imaging was arranged. All patients were imaged using US and X-ray KUBs. A contrast study of the lower or upper urinary tract to exclude functional or anatomical abnormalities was arranged when clinically indicated.

All relevant data were recorded on SPSS-21 for analysis. The stone size was entered as the largest dimension measured by the US and X-ray KUB. When there was a discrepancy in the measurement between the two methods, the largest diameter measured in either of them was used.

Computer software was used to randomize patients into two treatment groups. In the first group, patients were treated with pneumatic CL, whereas patients in the second were treated using laser CL. The patient's assignment into one of the treatment groups was recorded in the patient's medical record and disclosed to the treating surgeon on the morning of the operation.

All patients were fasted for 6–8 h and admitted to the hospital on the day of surgery. According to the hospital rules, all pediatric patients were treated at the start of the list and according to their age.

All procedures were conducted by one senior urologist utilizing general anesthesia while patients were in a semilithotomy position. A single prophylactic dose of intravenous antibiotic (cephazolin 30 mg/kg, unless urine culture and sensitivity or patient allergy profile dictate another antibiotic) was administered at time of anesthesia induction.

Initially, urethrocystoscopy was performed with an 8 Fr. Pediatric cystoscope to exclude urethral/bladder abnormalities and document the presence of the stones. A 9 Fr. semirigid ureteroscope was then used to pass the lithotripter through and fragment the stone (0.8 mm tip cystolithoclast, Karl Storz, or 365 µm quartz fiber Ho:YAG, CALCULASE II, Karl Storz). No energy was applied until the probe was clearly observed to be in contact with the stone. Pneumatic energy was applied in a pulsatile manner while laser was applied with 6–10 Hz, 1 J (for fragmentation), and 10–15 Hz, 0.5–0.8 J (for dusting). Normal saline was used for irrigation, and large stone fragments were extracted with a Storz grasper.

Stone fragmentation continued until stone-free status was achieved or it was not safe to continue because of severe hematuria impairing vision. Stone-free status was confirmed intraoperatively by comparing the stone fragments with the probe tip and postoperatively using US/X-ray KUB one week after the operation. All fragments larger than twice the probe tip were either fragmented more or removed with a stone grasper.

Operation time was calculated from the insertion of the ureteroscope for the first time to the removal of the last cystoscope/ureteroscope after stone fragments retrieval and/or washout.

An 8–12 Fr indwelling urethral catheter (IDC) was introduced at the end of the procedure and later patients were admitted into the ward and kept on oral paracetamol every 6 hours, with instructions for a trial of void (TOV) at 7 AM in the next morning. Patients were allowed to restart their oral intake once fully recovered from anesthesia, and no patient received IV fluid postoperatively. Outpatient follow-up continued for at least 6 months after discharge from the hospital. Children who failed the initial TOV were recatheterized and had their bladders examined by US to exclude presence of significant blood clots and then given a second TOV after 24 h. Any temperature greater than 37.5 °C was considered significant, and those patients were started on oral antibiotics after sending urine samples for culture and sensitivity. The degree of macroscopic hematuria was estimated visually; when it was more than a faint rose in color, it was considered significant and an indication to postpone patient discharge from hospital. Data were tabulated and analyzed statistically in SPSS-21 (Chicago, IL, USA). Qualitative data were expressed as percentages, and quantitative data were expressed as mean ± standard deviation (SD).

The primary outcome of the study was to compare the stone-free rates in the treatment group. The complication rate in both groups was compared also and regarded as a secondary outcome.

3. Results

A total of 73 children were diagnosed with bladder stones during the study period, but only 64 were enrolled in the study. Nine patients were excluded, five of them due to presence of urinary tract infection, three due to multiple stones and one due to neuropathic bladder.

Of the 64 children who completed the study, 33 were treated with pneumatic CL and 31 were treated with laser CL. Demographic and baseline parameters in both groups were comparable, as evident in Table 1. In regard to the diet status of the patients, all patients followed a Middle Eastern Iraqi diet, of which the main components are wheat, barley and rice, dairy products and red meat (lamb and beef).

Table 1. Demographics and clinical data in both treatment groups.

Postoperative Outcomes	Pneumatic Lithotripsy (n = 33)	Laser Lithotripsy (n = 31)	p-Value
Age (years) (mean ± SD)	4.2 ± 2.2	3.9 ± 2.1	0.62
Sex (M:F)	30:3	30:1	0.61
Stone size (mm) (mean ± SD)	15.9 ± 4.6	15.7 ± 5.2	0.87
Duration of operation in minutes (mean ± SD)	51.5 ± 17.2	74.5 ± 26.6	**0.001**
Residual stones	2 (6.1)	1 (3.2)	1.0
Severe hematuria	4 (12.1)	4 (12.9)	1.0
Urinary retention after removal of catheter	2 (6.1)	1 (3.2)	1.0
Recurrence	2 (6.1)	1 (3.2)	1.0
Postoperative infection	4 (12.1)	1 (3.2)	0.36
Extended hospitalization	16 (48.5)	5 (16.1)	**0.006**
More than one day of IDC	10 (30.0)	6 (19.3)	0.19
Requirement for more than one session	2 (6.1)	1 (3.2)	1.0
At least one positive adverse outcome	21 (63.6)	12 (38.7)	**0.046**

Values are shown as number of patients, with percentage in parentheses, unless otherwise indicated.

Regarding the operation outcomes and complications, the laser lithotripsy group had a significantly longer duration of operation (74.5 ± 26.6 min vs. 51.5 ± 17.2 min, $p = 0.001$), whereas a significantly greater proportion of patients required an extended hospital stay in the pneumatic lithotripsy group (48.5% vs. 16.1%, $p = 0.006$). Moreover, pneumatic lithotripsy was associated with a significantly greater risk of having at least one adverse effect (64% greater than that in the laser group). Of the 31 patients who were treated with laser CL, only five (16.12%) required more than one day of hospitalization and each of those five required only 2 days. On the other hand, for those who were treated with pneumatic CL, 16 (48.48%) required more than one day of hospitalization, with an average stay of 2.64 days (eight patients for 2 days, five for 3 days and three for 4 days).

No significant difference was found between the two treatment groups in relation to stone clearance rates and all other studied adverse outcomes, as described in Table 1. Hematuria was found in four patients in each group (12%), and none of the patients required transfusion. No patient from those who had significant hematuria that delayed IDC removal and TOV was found to have a significant intravesical blood clot that required washout or a further delay of TOV.

Two patients in the pneumatic CL group and one in the laser CL group had significant residual stones and required a second procedure to clear the stone. All three patients had severe hematuria by the end of the procedure, which significantly impaired visualization.

In long-term follow-up, no patients in either group developed symptoms or signs suggestive of urethral stricture that required further investigation. Moreover, two patients re-presented with recurrent bladder stones in the pneumatic CL group and one did in the laser CL group.

A Mann–Whitney U test was used to analyze the scores of adverse outcomes in the two groups, and the difference was found not to be significant. In addition, a larger stone size was found to be associated with having at least one adverse outcome in both groups (Table 2).

Table 2. Differences in mean stone size between patients with at least one adverse outcome and those without adverse outcomes in both groups.

	Pneumatic Lithotripsy		Laser Lithotripsy	
	At Least One Adverse Outcome		At Least One Adverse Outcome	
	Negative	Positive	Negative	Positive
Mean stone size (mm)	13.1	17.5	12.4	21.0
Stone size range (mm)	(10–18)	(11–31)	(10–17)	(15–30)
SD	2.4	4.8	2.2	4.0
SE	0.70	1.04	0.51	1.15
n	12	21	19	12
p (t-test, negative vs. positive)	0.005		<0.001	

A multiple regression model was created and found to predict the risk of developing at least one adverse outcome with an accuracy of 84.4%. According to this model, pneumatic lithotripsy was associated with a significant increase in the risk of developing at least one adverse postoperative outcome (5.7 times that of the laser lithotripsy group) after adjustment for the possible confounding effects of age and stone size (Table 3). Age was not significantly associated with the risk of developing adverse outcomes (Table 3).

Table 3. Multiple regression model of the risk of developing at least one adverse outcome as the dependent variable.

	Partial OR	95% Confidence Interval OR	p-Value
Pneumatic lithotripsy compared with laser lithotripsy	5.7	(1.17–28)	0.031
Age	1.14	(0.81–1.59)	0.46 [NS]
Stone size (mm)	1.75	(1.33–2.29)	<0.001
Constant	0.000	(0–0)	<0.001

NS: nonsignificant; OR: odds ratio. Overall predictive accuracy = 84.4%. p (model) ≤ 0.001.

4. Discussion

Transurethral cystolitholapaxy and CL have been considered the first-line treatments for bladder stones in adults for decades; however, the use of these techniques in children was delayed for many years, during which open CL and percutaneous CL were the first-line treatment choices. These two surgical techniques are associated with significant morbidity, including scar formation, prolonged catheterization and longer hospital stays. Bowel injury is a more serious complication specific to percutaneous CL.

Later, the availability of pediatric cystoscopes and ureteroscopes, as well as highly effective intracorporeal lithotripsy devices with miniprobes, enabled the feasibility of transurethral CL in children [3,9,10,15]. Currently, pneumatic, laser and, to a lesser extent, electrohydraulic lithotripters are used to fragment stones in children [16]. Recent advances in robotic surgery will open the doors for even less invasive robotic-assisted removal of bladder stones in pediatric patients [12–14].

The safety and efficacy of pneumatic lithotripters in treating bladder stones in children were tested and reported by many authors following their initial use by Shokier [3,9,14,17]. Ho:YAG lasers enabled a major breakthrough in the management of stone disease in general. These lasers are safe and effective and can fragment many types of stones [10,17].

Each of these two lithotripter types has pros and cons. Pneumatic lithotripter probes are relatively inexpensive, and the energy generators are easy to maintain. The main problem associated with the use of pneumatic lithotripters is stone migration, owing to the ballistic mechanism used to fragment stones. Laser lithotripters, in contrast, are much more expensive. The probes are usually disposable, and the laser generators are costly to maintain. Laser, however, has the advantages of being able to fragment stones into submillimeter pieces without significant stone migration and of eliminating the need to use graspers to extract larger stone fragments [18].

This prospective study aimed to compare the safety and efficacy of pneumatic and laser lithotripters in treating children with bladder stones. The patient age, sex and stone size were comparable between the two treatment groups and were not expected to confound the analysis.

Because operation time is an important factor in any surgical procedure, we compared the time required to fragment stones with pneumatic and laser CL. Laser stone fragmentation required significantly longer durations (74.5 vs. 51.5 min). Gangkak and coworkers reported no significant difference in operation time between laser and pneumatic lithotripsy (36.6 vs. 35.5) [17]. They also reported a much shorter operation time than that in our study. This discrepancy might be explained by our limited experience in using laser lithotripsy, given that this method was newly introduced to our center, as well as by our practice of reusing the laser fibers to conserve our limited resources, thus potentially decreasing the laser fiber efficiency.

In comparing the outcomes of surgery, we found that the two groups had comparable stone-free rates and postoperative complications. A Mann–Whitney U test used to count the scores of adverse outcomes did not indicate any significant differences between the two groups. The only significant difference observed was that patients treated with pneumatic lithotripsy required longer hospital stays than those treated with laser lithotripsy. Only five patients (16.1%) treated with laser lithotripsy required an extended hospital stay, and all of them required one additional day. In the pneumatic lithotripsy group, in contrast, almost half the patients required an extension of their hospital stay (16 patients, 48.48%). The average hospital stays for patients who required an extended stay in the laser CL group was 2 days, compared to 2.68 days in the pneumatic CL group.

Of the 16 patients who required extended hospital stays in the pneumatic CL group, eight patients had 2 days of admission, five patients had 3 days and three patients had 4 days. Reasons for the longer-than-planned hospital stay were hematuria in four patients, failed TOV in two patients, infection in four patients and pain or parents' anxiety in six patients. Apart from parents' anxiety, all other causes of extended hospital stay were attributed to the surgery itself. Postoperative pain score was difficult to appreciate or measure in children, and this was the reason behind excluding pain as a postoperative complication to measure and compare in both treatment groups.

In a comparison of overall outcomes, the risk of having at least one adverse outcome was higher in the pneumatic lithotripsy group ($p = 0.046$).

The mean stone size in patients with at least one adverse outcome was significantly higher in both treatment groups and can be considered an independent predictor of adverse outcomes. Aboulela and colleagues divided patients into two groups according to stone size and treated them with laser lithotripsy and found that the operation time and complication rate significantly differed between groups [19]. A similar finding was reported by Abdul Rasheed and coworkers in patients treated with pneumatic lithotripsy [8]. The authors, however, reported a greater overall rate of complications, which may have been associated with the urethral dilation performed at the start of the procedure in that study.

The rate of urinary tract infection after pneumatic lithotripsy was four times higher than that after laser lithotripsy (4 (12.1%) vs. 1 (3.2%)), but this difference was not statistically significant ($p = 0.36$). This result may be associated with previous recurrent use of stone graspers to clear out larger stone fragments in the patients treated with pneumatic lithotripsy.

To identify factors that independently predicted the outcome, we created a multiple regression model and found that pneumatic lithotripsy and stone size were the only two factors that independently predicted the outcome. Compared with laser lithotripsy, pneumatic lithotripsy increased the risk of at least one adverse outcome by 5.7 times. The model also showed that every 1 mm increase in stone size was associated with a 75% increase in the chance of an adverse outcome. Patient age and sex of the patient were not found to be independent factors affecting the surgery outcomes.

No long-term complications were found in any of the treated patients in terms of urethral stricture or chronic lower urinary tract symptoms. Similar results were reported by most previous studies [9,10,15,17,19]. Abdul Rasheed and colleagues also reported a 3.5% rate of urethral stricture after pneumatic lithotripsy, which again might have been associated with the urethral dilation that was performed. Al-Marhoon and associates compared G and pneumatic lithotripsy to open cystolithotomy. One of their patients treated with pneumatic lithotripsy had a urethral rupture with extravasation and later developed urethral stricture [20]. In their conclusion, the authors recommend the use of laser fibers through a ureteroscope to reduce the risk of urethral injury. Javanmard and colleagues compared transurethral laser lithotriopsy with open and percutaneous cystolithotomy in treating bladder stones in children and described laser as a safe, effective and minimally invasive treatment option [21].

One of the study limitations is stone composition, which is another factor that must be considered. Some stones are difficult to fragment and take too long to be destroyed. Unfortunately, our study, like most of the studies related to this topic, does not report on the stone composition. In a trial to overcome this issue, we performed an X-ray KUB to check for stone radiopacity. However, this, unfortunately, was not very helpful, as only four stones in both groups were radiopaque.

In our center, the laser machine was introduced only recently, and we, therefore, face technical and financial hurdles in maintaining the energy generator and the laser fibers. Because our public hospital has a high workload and limited resources, we must consider these hurdles when choosing treatment modalities, despite the apparent superiority of laser over pneumatic lithotripsy.

5. Conclusions

Pneumatic and laser lithotripsy are equal with regard to stone clearance rate. However, pneumatic lithotripsy has a shorter operating time, longer hospital stays and a more adverse effect. Laser lithotripsy appears to be relatively superior to pneumatic lithotripsy in terms of being associated with fewer complications, but its cost might limit its use. In choosing the treatment modality, stone size is the most important factor to consider in cases in which complications are expected.

Author Contributions: Conceptualization, Z.H.A. and S.A.M.; methodology, Z.H.A. and S.A.M.; software, S.A.M.; validation, Z.H.A.; data curation, Z.H.A. and S.A.M.; writing—original draft preparation, Z.H.A.; writing—review and editing, Z.H.A. and S.A.M. visualization, Z.H.A. and S.A.M.; supervision, Z.H.A. and S.A.M. All authors have read and agreed to the published version of the manuscript.

Funding: This research received no external funding.

Institutional Review Board Statement: The study was conducted in accordance with the Declaration of Helsinki and approved by the Ethics Committee of University of Anbar with an ethical code of 128 EA.

Informed Consent Statement: Informed consent was obtained from all subjects involved in the study.

Data Availability Statement: Data can be obtained from the corresponding author based on a reasonable request.

Conflicts of Interest: The authors declare no conflict of interest.

References

1. Colin, B.A. The epidemiology, formation, composition and medical management of idiopathic stone disease. *Curr. Opin. Urol.* **1993**, *33*, 16–22.
2. Rizvi, S.A.H.; Naqvi, S.A.A.; Hussain, Z.; Hashmi, A.; Hussain, M.; Zafar, M.N.; Mehdi, H.; Khalid, R. The management of stone disease. *BJU Int.* **2002**, *896*, 2–8. [CrossRef] [PubMed]
3. Hussain, M. Endemic bladder calculi in children. What is current position? *J. Nephrol. Urol. Transpl.* **2001**, *21*, 1–2.
4. Cicione, A.; De Nunzio, C.; Manno, S.; Damiano, R.; Posti, A.; Lima, E.; Tubaro, A.; Balloni, F. Bladder stone management: An update. *Minerva Urol. Nefrol.* **2018**, *70*, 53–65. [CrossRef] [PubMed]
5. Ali, S.H.; Rifat, U.N. Etiological and clinical patterns of childhood urolithiasis in Iraq. *Pediatr. Nephrol.* **2005**, *201*, 453–457. [CrossRef] [PubMed]
6. Papatsoris, A.G.; Varkarakis, I.; Dellis, A. Bladder lithiasis: From open surgery to lithotripsy. *Urology* **2006**, *341*, 63–67. [CrossRef] [PubMed]
7. Mahran, M.R.; Dawaba, M.S. Cystitholapaxy versus cystolithotomy in children. *J. Endourol.* **2000**, *144*, 23–26. [CrossRef] [PubMed]
8. Abdul, R.S.; Ghulam, S.S.; Abdul, H.; Shaikh, A. Endoscopic treatment of vesical calculi in children. *RMJ* **2010**, *35*, 15–18.
9. Shokier, A.A. Transurethral cystitholapaxy in children. *J. Endourol.* **1994**, *81*, 57–60. [CrossRef] [PubMed]
10. Esposito, C.; Autorino, G.; Masieri, L.; Castagnetti, M.; Del Conte, F.; Coppola, V.; Cerulo, M.; Crocetto, F.; Escolino, M. Minimally Invasive Management of Bladder Stones in Children. *Front. Pediatr.* **2021**, *86*, 18756. [CrossRef] [PubMed]
11. Esposito, C.; Masieri, L.; Blanc, T.; Lendvay, T.; Escolino, M. Robot-assisted laparoscopic surgery for treatment of urinary tract stones in children: Report of a multicenter international experience. *Urolithiasis* **2021**, *49*, 575–583. [CrossRef] [PubMed]
12. Scarcella, S.; Tiroli, M.; Torino, G.; Mariscoli, F.; Cobellis, G.; Galosi, A.B. Combined treatment of ureteropelvic junction obstruction and renal calculi with robot-assisted laparoscopic pyeloplasty and laser lithotripsy in children: Case report and non-systematic review of the literature. *Int. J. Med. Robot.* **2021**, *17*, e2246. [CrossRef] [PubMed]
13. Esposito, C.; Autorino, G.; Castagnetti, M.; Cerulo, M.; Coppola, V.; Cardone, R.; Esposito, G.; Borgogni, R.; Escolino, M. Robotics and future technical developments in pediatric urology. *Semin. Pediatr. Surg.* **2021**, *30*, 151082. [CrossRef] [PubMed]
14. Ramakrishnan, P.A.; Medhat, M.; Al-Bulushi, Y.H. Holmium laser cystolithotripsy in children: Initial experience. *Can. J. Urol.* **2005**, *122*, 880–886.
15. Isen, K.; Em, S.; Kilic, V.; Utku, V.; Bogatekin, S.; Ergin, H. Management of bladder stones with pneumatic lithotripsy using a ureteroscope in children. *J. Endourol.* **2008**, *221*, 037–040. [CrossRef] [PubMed]
16. Kauer, P.C.; Laguna, M.P.; Aliviazatos, G. Present practice and treatment strategies in endourological stone management: Results of a surgery of the European Society of Uro-technology (ESUT). *Eur. Urol.* **2005**, *481*, 82–88.
17. Gangkak, G.; Sher, S.Y.; Vinay, T.; Nachiket, V.; Deepak, J. Pneumatic cystolithotripsy versus holmium:yag laser cystolithotripsy in the treatment of pediatric bladder stones: A prospective randomized study. *Pediatr. Surg. Int.* **2016**, *326*, 9–14. [CrossRef] [PubMed]
18. Brian, R.M.; James, E.L. Surgical management of upper urinary tract calculi. In *Campbell's Urology*, 10th ed.; Walsh, P.C., Retik, A.B., Vaughan, E.D., Eds.; WB Saunders: Philadelphia, PA, USA, 2012; pp. 1382–1388.
19. Aboulela, W.; ElSheemy, M.S.; Shoukry, A.I.; Shouman, A.M.; ElShenoufy, A.; Daw, K. Transurethral holmium laser cystolithotripsy in children: Single center experience. *J. Endourol.* **2014**, *29*, 661–665. [CrossRef] [PubMed]
20. Al-Marhoon, M.S.; Sarhan, O.M.; Awad, B.A.; Helmy, T.; Ghali, A.; Dawaba, M.S. Comparison of endourological and open cystolithotomy in the management of bladder stones in children. *J. Urol.* **2009**, *1812*, 648–688. [CrossRef] [PubMed]
21. Javanmard, B.; Fallah Karkan, M.; Razzaghi, M.R.; Ghiasy, S.; Ranjbar, A.; Rahavian, A. Surgical Management of Vesical Stones in Children: A Comparison Between Open Cystolithotomy, Percutaneous Cystolithotomy and Transurethral Cystolithotripsy with Holmium-YAG Laser. *J. Lasers Med. Sci.* **2018**, *9*, 183–187. [CrossRef] [PubMed]

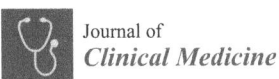

Review

Catheter-Associated Urinary Infections and Consequences of Using Coated versus Non-Coated Urethral Catheters—Outcomes of a Systematic Review and Meta-Analysis of Randomized Trials

Vineet Gauhar [1], Daniele Castellani [2,*], Jeremy Yuen-Chun Teoh [3], Carlotta Nedbal [2], Giuseppe Chiacchio [2], Andrew T. Gabrielson [4], Flavio Lobo Heldwein [5], Marcelo Langer Wroclawski [6,7], Jean de la Rosette [8], Rodrigo Donalisio da Silva [9], Andrea Benedetto Galosi [2] and Bhaskar Kumar Somani [10]

1. Department of Urology, Ng Teng Fong General Hospital (NUHS), Singapore 609606, Singapore; vineetgaauhaar@gmail.com
2. Urology Unit, Azienda Ospedaliero-Universitaria Ospedali Riuniti di Ancona, Università Politecnica delle Marche, 60126 Ancona, Italy; carlottanedbal@gmail.com (C.N.); gipeppo1@gmail.com (G.C.); andreabenedetto.galosi@ospedaliriuniti.marche.it (A.B.G.)
3. S.H.Ho Urology Centre, Department of Surgery, The Chinese University of Hong Kong, Hong Kong, China; jeremyteoh@surgery.cuhk.edu.hk
4. Brady Urological Institute, Johns Hopkins Medical Institutions, Baltimore, MD 21287, USA; andrewtgabe@gmail.com
5. Department of Urology, Universidade Federal de Santa Catarina, Florianópolis 88040-900, Brazil; flavio.lobo@gmail.com
6. Hospital Israelita Albert Einstein, São Paulo 05652-900, Brazil; urologia.marcelo@gmail.com
7. Beneficência Portuguesa de São Paulo (BP), São Paulo 01323-001, Brazil
8. Department of Urology, Medipol Mega University Hospital, Istanbul Medipol University, 34214 Istanbul, Turkey; j.j.delarosette@gmail.com
9. Division of Urology, Denver Health Medical Center, University of Colorado, Denver, CO 80204, USA; rodrigo.donalisiodasilva@dhha.org
10. Department of Urology, University Hospitals Southampton, NHS Trust, Southampton SO16 6YD, UK; bhaskarsomani@yahoo.com
* Correspondence: castellanidaniele@gmail.com; Tel.: +39-71-5963367

Abstract: Coated urethral catheters were introduced in clinical practice to reduce the risk of catheter-acquired urinary tract infection (CAUTI). We aimed to systematically review the incidence of CAUTI and adverse effects in randomized clinical trials of patients requiring indwelling bladder catheterization by comparing coated vs. non-coated catheters. This review was performed according to the 2020 PRISMA framework. The incidence of CAUTI and catheter-related adverse events was evaluated using the Cochran–Mantel–Haenszel method with a random-effects model and reported as the risk ratio (RR), 95% CI, and p-values. Significance was set at $p < 0.05$ and a 95% CI. Twelve studies including 36,783 patients were included for meta-analysis. There was no significant difference in the CAUTI rate between coated and non-coated catheters (RR 0.87 95% CI 0.75–1.00, $p = 0.06$). Subgroup analysis demonstrated that the risk of CAUTI was significantly lower in the coated group compared with the non-coated group among patients requiring long-term catheterization (>14 days) (RR 0.82 95% CI 0.68–0.99, $p = 0.04$). There was no difference between the two groups in the incidence of the need for catheter exchange or the incidence of lower urinary tract symptoms after catheter removal. The benefit of coated catheters in reducing CAUTI risk among patients requiring long-term catheterization should be balanced against the increased direct costs to health care systems when compared to non-coated catheters.

Keywords: urinary catheters; catheters; indwelling; catheter-related infections

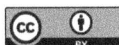

1. Introduction

The word catheter is derived from the ancient Greek *kathiénai*, literally meaning "to thrust into" or "to send down" [1]. In use for more than 3500 years, urethral catheters are a bane and boon for patients and urologists alike as they may pose a risk to patients requiring long-term catheterization. The most common problems include hematuria, catheter encrustation requiring frequent catheter exchange, and catheter-acquired urinary tract infection (CAUTI).

With technical advancements in bioengineering and materials science, several types of indwelling catheters were developed to prevent CAUTI and improve patient tolerance. Coating agents were added to catheter surfaces to improve antimicrobial proprieties and to provide robust antibiofilm/antimicrobial activity, without causing an increase in patient discomfort [2,3]. Coated catheters can be divided into two types: those coated in antifouling materials, and those impregnated with bactericidal molecules.

Antifouling substances do not kill the bacteria but rather perturb their ability to colonize surfaces, preventing the formation of biofilms in the bladder or on the catheter surface. The most common antifouling materials are hydrogel and polytetrafluoroethylene (PTFE). Hydrogel catheters may reduce encrustation via forming hydration layers on the catheter surface; however, studies have demonstrated a similar incidence of nosocomial CAUTI and a higher rate of blockage when compared to standard silicone catheters [4]. PTFE-coated catheters seem to be more suitable candidates to inhibit biofilm formation because of their low coefficient of friction. Unfortunately, studies have demonstrated that PTFE-coated catheters are not superior to hydrogel or standard silicone catheters in preventing CAUTI [2].

Catheters can also be coated with antimicrobial agents such as metal ions (i.e., silver, gold, and/or palladium), antibiotics, and nitrofurazone. Among bactericidal-coated catheters, silver-coated catheters are the most popular and widely tested catheters. The release of silver ions into the bladder induces oxidative stress and disrupts bacteria membrane and proteins, but antimicrobial efficacy may vary with the silver-coated substance used. Although in vitro and in vivo studies have shown great efficacy in preventing infections [5], these have not necessarily translated to clear benefits in clinical trials [6].

Antibiotic-coated catheters are less frequently used, especially with the increased frequency of having multi-drug-resistant bacteria [2]. Nitrofurazone was a promising coating agent in in vivo and in vitro studies, but it was not efficient in preventing infections in clinical studies and caused patient discomfort [7].

This study aimed to systematically review the incidence of CAUTI and its adverse effects in randomized clinical trials of patients requiring indwelling bladder catheterization (transurethral or suprapubic) by comparing coated vs. non-coated catheters.

2. Materials and Methods

2.1. Aim of This Review

The present study aims to systematically review the incidence of CAUTI in patients requiring indwelling bladder catheterization by comparing coated vs. non-coated catheters. The primary outcome was the CAUTI rate between the two types of catheters. The secondary outcomes were the CAUTI rate according to catheterization time (cut-off: 14 days) and the rate of catheter-related adverse events (i.e., hematuria, need for catheter exchange or catheter removal, urinary symptoms after catheter removal). Additionally a cost-effectiveness analysis was performed.

2.2. Literature Search

This review was performed according to the 2020 Preferred Reporting Items for Systematic Reviews and Meta-Analyses (PRISMA) framework. A broad literature search was performed on 1 May 2022, using MEDLINE, EMBASE, and Cochrane Central Register of Controlled Trials. Medical Subject Heading (MeSH) terms and keywords such as (urinary tract infection OR infections OR sepsis) AND (short term OR long OR indwelling) AND (standard urethral catheter OR impregnated urethral catheter OR silicone OR hydrogel OR antibiotic coated OR silver-impregnated) were used. The search was restricted to English papers only. No date limits were imposed. Pediatric and animal studies were excluded. The review protocol was submitted for registration in PROSPERO (receipt #332889).

2.3. Selection Criteria

The Patient Intervention Comparison Outcome Study (PICOS) model was used to frame and answer the clinical question. P: adults requiring bladder catheterization; Intervention: coated catheters; Comparison: non-coated catheters; Outcome: CAUTI and catheter-related adverse effects; Study type: prospective and randomized studies. Patients were assigned to two groups according to the type of catheter (coated vs. non-coated catheters).

2.4. Study Screening and Selection

Two independent authors screened all retrieved records through Covidence Systematic Review Management® (Veritas Health Innovation, Melbourne, Australia). Discrepancies were solved by a third author. Studies were included based on PICOS eligibility criteria. Only prospective and randomized studies were accepted. Meeting abstracts, retrospective, and prospective nonrandomized studies were excluded. Case reports, reviews, letters to the editor, and editorials were excluded. The full text of the screened papers was selected if found relevant to the purpose of this study.

2.5. Statistical Analysis

The incidence of CAUTI and catheter-related adverse effects was evaluated using the Cochran–Mantel–Haenszel method with a random-effects model and reported as the risk ratio (RR), 95% CI, and *p*-values. For studies with 3 groups of patients, intervention groups were combined to create a single pair-wise comparison [8]. Analyses were two tailed and significance was set at $p < 0.05$ and a 95% CI. Study heterogeneity was assessed utilizing the I^2 value. Substantial heterogeneity was defined as an I^2 value > 50%. Meta-analysis was performed using Review Manager (RevMan) 5.4 software by Cochrane Collaboration. The quality assessment of the included studies was performed using RoB 2 [9].

3. Results

The literature search retrieved 2689 studies. After eliminating 297 duplicates, 2392 studies were left for screening. Another 2326 papers were further excluded against the title and abstract screening because they were unrelated to the purpose of this review. The full texts of the remaining 66 studies were screened and 54 papers were further excluded. Finally, 12 studies were accepted and included for meta-analysis. Figure 1 shows the PRISMA flow diagram.

3.1. Study Characteristics and Quality Assessment

Twelve prospective, randomized studies compared coated vs. non-coated catheters in patients requiring an indwelling catheter [7,10–20]. No study with a suprapubic catheter was retrieved. Study characteristics are summarized in Table 1. Only one study had catheters with antibacterial/antifouling coating (i.e., hydrogel) [16] and the other 11 had catheters coated with bactericidal molecules, i.e., pure silver ions [7,10,12,13,18], noble ions (silver, gold, palladium) [14], or silver ions mixed with hydrogel [19], nitrofurazone [7,11,15,17], and a polymer of zinc oxide bonded carbon nanotube [20]. There were 36,783 patients included in 12 studies: 19,404 patients in the coated catheter group and 17,379 in the non-coated catheter group.

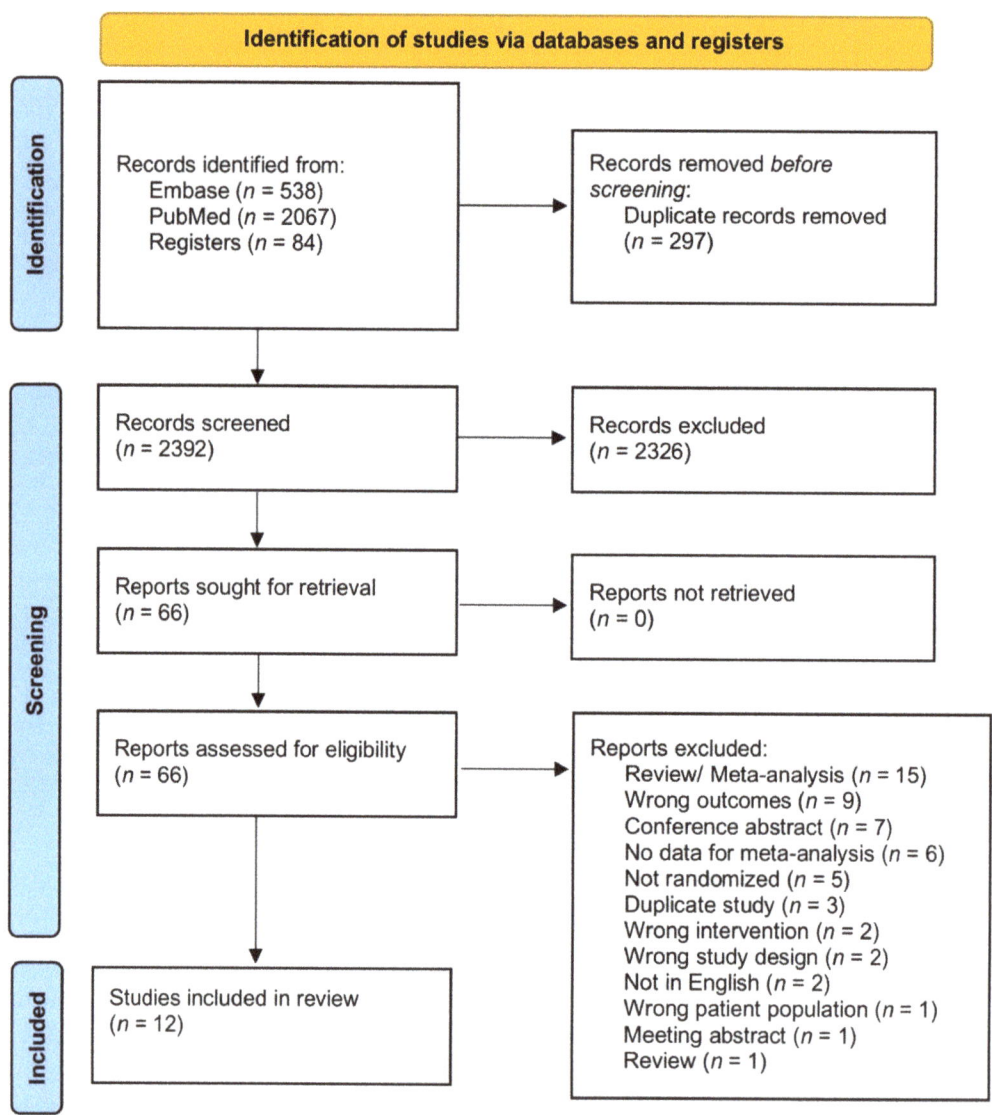

Figure 1. PRISMA diagram of this study.

Table 2 shows data on pathogen species isolated in urine culture. The most common detected pathogens were *Escheria coli*, *Enterococcus*, *Pseudomonas* spp., *Klebsiella* spp., Gram-positive cocci, including *Staphylococcus aureus*, followed by *Candida* spp. and *Yeasts*. Polymicrobial infections were uncommon.

Table 1. Characteristics of the included studies. NA: not available. UTI: urinary tract infections. SCI: spinal cord injury.

	Inclusion Criteria	Exclusion Criteria	Length of Follow Up	Type of Coated Catheter	Number of Patients Included in Coated Catheter	Mean Age (Standard Deviation) in Coated Group	Type of Non-Coated Catheter	Number of Patients Included in Non-Coated Catheter	Mean Age (Standard Deviation) in Non-Coated Group	Catheter Duration (Days)
Akcam 2019 [10]	Patients admitted to the intensive care unit and anticipated to require long-term urinary catheterization	Patients with any infectious disease on admission or with pyuria/bacteriuria in the first urine specimen collected following catheter placement	Until discharge of patients	Silver-coated silicone catheters	28	70.61 (NA)	silicone catheters	26	69.23 (NA)	NA
Bonfill 2017 [8]	Patients with traumatic or medical SCI requiring an indwelling urinary catheter for at least 7 days	Patients with demonstrable UTI at the time of inclusion; taking antibiotic treatment at the time of inclusion or for any infectious condition or within 7 days before inclusion	12 months	Silver alloy catheters	243	55.30 (16.35)	silicone catheters	246	57.25 (16.32)	27 in coated 28 in non-coated
Erickson 2008 [6]	Men undergoing urethral reconstruction	None	20 months	Hydrogel-coated latex foley	42	40 (NA)	silicone catheters	43	43 (NA)	14–21
Johnson 1990 [3]	Patients with a steady catheter that was expected to remain indwelling for at least 24 h	UTI at enrollment	16 months	Silicone catheter coated with a layer of silicone elastomer containing micronized silver oxide	207	50 (NA)	silicone catheters	208	47 (NA)	3 in coated 4 in non-coated
Karchmer 2000 [2]	Hospitalized patients with vesical catheters	Pediatric, obstetrics, gynecology, and psychiatry wards excluded	12 months	Silver-alloy, hydrogel-coated latex catheters	13,945	NA	silicone catheters	13,933	NA	>7 days
Lee 2004 [7]	Patients who were catheterized for more than 24 h	conditions such as silicone sensitivity, nitrofurazone or nitrofurantoin sensitivity, pregnancy, lactating, hospitalization for more than 7 days, and having urinary diseases; positive urine culture result before catheter insertion or when the catheter was removed within 24 h of insertion	7 days	Release nitrofurazone foley catheter	92	55.3	silicone catheters	85	54.1	3.9–4.4
Menezes 2019 [11]	urethral catheterization for kidney transplantation with a living donor	asymptomatic bacteriuria or urinary tract infection at baseline, deceased kidney transplant donors, hypersensitivity to nitrofurantoin, pregnancy	22 months	Nitrofural-impregnated silicone catheter	88	38.4 (NA)	silicone catheters	88	39.6 (NA)	5.1

Table 1. Cont.

	Inclusion Criteria	Exclusion Criteria	Length of Follow Up	Type of Coated Catheter	Number of Patients Included in Coated Catheter	Mean Age (Standard Deviation) in Coated Group	Type of Non-Coated Catheter	Number of Patients Included in Non-Coated Catheter	Mean Age (Standard Deviation) in Non-Coated Group	Catheter Duration (Days)
Pickard 2012 [7]	Adults undergoing urethral catheterization for an anticipated duration of up to 14 days (including people with diabetes and individuals treated with immunosuppressive drugs)	Symptomatic urinary tract infection at baseline, urological procedures in the previous 7 days, or allergies to catheter materials	39 months	(1) Silver alloy-coated latex catheter (2) Nitrofural-impregnated silicone catheter	(1) 2097 (2) 2153	(1) 59 (16) (2) 59 (16)	standard polytetrafluoroethylene (PTFE)-coated latex catheter	2144	59 (16)	2 (1–3)
Stensballe 2007 [15]	trauma patients who needed a urinary catheter and were admitted directly from the accident scene to the Trauma Center	HIV infection; preinjury treatment with corticosteroids; pregnancy; primary burn injury; and unattainable signed informed consent	24 months	Nitrofurazone-impregnated catheter	106	41 (NA)	silicone catheters	106	43 (NA)	2 (0–7)
Stenzelius 2011 [14]	patients undergoing elective orthopedic surgery	recent (within 3 weeks) use of a urinary catheter or a recent history of UTI, previous radiation therapy over the lower pelvis, latex allergy, cognitive impairment, or difficulties in understanding the Swedish language	2–7 days	Noble metal alloy-coated latex catheter	222	67.6 (12)	silicone catheters	217	66.7 (12.8)	2
Tae 2022 [20]	Patients underwent radical cystectomy with neobladder cause of invasive bladder cancer	Malnutrition, active infection, immunodeficiency, allergy to components	NA	Carbon nanotube and ZnO-bonded CNT	41	65.22 (10.25)	silicone catheters	44	65.36 (8.56)	14 + or − 1
Thibon 2000 [19]	Patients in neurosurgery ICU required catheter during admission for more than three days and had to stay in hospital for at least 10 days after the insertion of a urinary catheter	urinary tract infection or inflammation of the perineum or penis before catheter insertion, allergy to hydrogel or silver salts, contraindications for catheterization, urinary tract catheter insertion during the 48 h before inclusion, antibiotic treatment for urinary tractinfection and other types of urinary tract intervention (prostate, bladder)	24 months	Hydrogel and silver salt-coated catheter	90	59.8 (17.1)	silicone catheters	109	60.5 (15.5)	10

Table 2. Pathogens isolated in urine cultures.

	Pathogen Species in Urine Culture	Difference in Urine Culture between Coated and Non-Coated Catheters
Akcam 2019 [10]	The most commonly detected agent, at 11/25 (44%), was Escherichia coli (44%), Enterococcus spp. (20%), Klebsiella pneumonia (8%), Pseudomonas spp. (8%), Acinetobacter spp. (8%), Enterobacter cloacae (4%), Proteus mirabilis (4%) and Candida spp. (4%). Second species were grown in four of the specimens: Enterococcus spp. was isolated in three specimens, and E. cloacae in one of the specimens	E. coli grew in 26.9%, and microorganisms other than E. coli in 19.3% of the subjects using normal catheters, while E. coli grew in 14.3% and other microorganisms in 32.1% of the patients using silver-coated catheters
Bonfill 2017 [18]	Not reported in full	One patient, pertaining to the group with SAC urinary catheter, developed a urinary septic shock caused by Proteus mirabilis. Another patient, pertaining to the group of standard urinary catheter, developed a urinary sepsis caused by Escherichia coli and P. mirabilis
Erickson 2008 [16]	Not reported	Not reported
Johnson 1990 [13]	Coagulase-negative staphylococci, Enterococcus species, Escherichia coli, Proteus mirabilis, Pseudomonas species, Yeast other	No difference
Karchmer 2000 [2]	Escherichia coli (18.4%), Escherichia faecalis (16.9%), Candida albicans (13.4%), and Pseudomonas aeruginosa (11.7%), Yeast (26.2%), Gram-positive cocci, including Staphylococcus aureus, coagulase-negative staphylococci, and enterococci (28%)	There were no statistically significant differences in the proportion of infections attributed to different organisms following use of silver-coated and uncoated catheters
Lee 2004 [17]	Enterococcus species (22.5%), Staphylococcus (15%), Pseudomonas species (30%), StenotrophomonasMaltophilia (10%), others (Acinetobacter calcoaceticus–baumannii complex, A. luoffi, Citrobacter freundii, Enterobacter cloacae, Nonfermenting Gram–negative Bacillus, Pasteurella multocida, Burkholderia cepacia, B. pseudomallei, Chryseobacterium meningosepticum 15%). Mixed infection was observed in five patients	StenotrophomonasMaltophilia was not isolated in patients with non-coated catheters
Menezes 2019 [11]	Gram-negative bacilli (95.24%) and Escherichia coli was the most frequently isolated microorganism (47.62%). Among the isolates of E. coli and Klebsiella pneumoniae, 25% had an extended spectrum beta-lactamase producing profile, and 12.5% of the K pneumonie strains were carbapenem resistant	No evidence of enhanced antimicrobial resistance with the employment of the Nitrofurazone-coated urinary catheter
Pickard 2012 [7]	Not reported	Not reported
Stensballe 2007 [15]	Enterococcus species, Escherichia coli, Candida species, Coagulase-negative staphylococci, Corynebacterium species, Pseudomonas aeruginosa, polymicrobial	Nitrofurantoin resistance was found in 3 isolates in the nitrofurazone group (1 with Pseudomonas aeruginosa and 2 with Candida species) compared with 7 in the silicone group (1 with Enterobacter species, 5 with Candida species, and 1 with Enterobacter species and Candida species)
Stenzelius 2011 [14]	Not reported	Not reported
Tae 2022 [20]	Enterococcus faecalis, Proteus, Pseudomonas aeruginosa, Yeast, Streptococcus species, Klebsiella pneumoniae, methicillin-resistant Staphylococcus aureus	Coated: 19 positive cultures. Non-coated: 22 positive cultures Enterococcus faecalis: coated 8; non-coated 11 Pseudomonas aeruginosa: coated 4; non-coated 4 Yeast: coated 3; non-coated 2 Streptococcus species: coated 2; non-coated 4 Klebsiella pneumoniae: coated 1; non-coated 2 methicillin-resistant Staphylococcus aureus: coated 1; non-coated 1
Thibon 2000 [19]	Escherichia coli, Proteus, Pseudomonas, Enterobacter cloacae, Yeasts, coagulase negative staphylococci, enterococci, others	There was no significant difference between the types of organism identified with the two types of catheter

Figure 2 shows the details of quality assessment in the included studies. Six studies showed a low overall risk of bias and the remaining six demonstrated some concerns. The most common reason for bias arose from the randomization process, followed by bias due to missing outcome data.

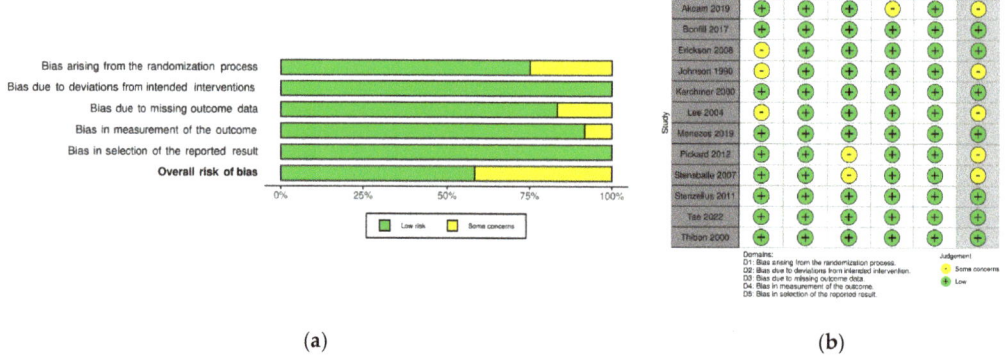

(a)   (b)

Figure 2. Risk of bias of the included study (Rob2): (**a**) review authors' judgments about each risk of bias item presented as percentages across all included studies; (**b**) review authors' judgments about each risk of bias item for each included study.

3.2. Meta-Analysis of CAUTI

Meta-analysis from 12 studies (19,328 cases in the coated and 17,287 cases in the non-coated group) showed that the risk of CAUTI did not differ significantly between the groups (RR 0.87 95% CI 0.75–1.00, $p = 0.06$) (Figure 3). There was no significant heterogeneity among the studies ($I^2 = 22\%$). Subgroup analysis for catheter dwelling time demonstrated that the risk of CAUTI was significantly lower in the coated group compared with the non-coated group (RR 0.82 95% CI 0.68–0.99, $p = 0.04$). Only one study reported the rate of sepsis and another the rate of cystitis, making meta-analysis not feasible.

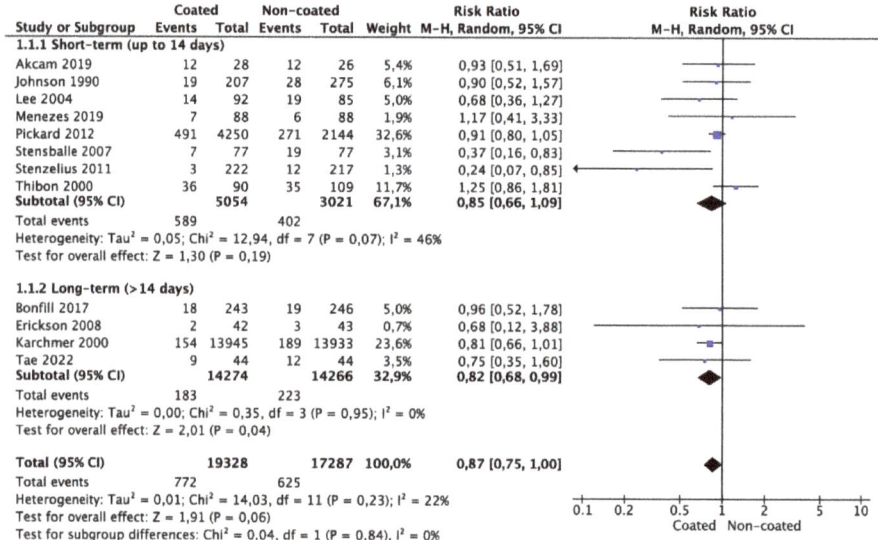

Figure 3. Meta-analysis of CAUTI incidence.

3.3. Meta-Analysis of Need for Catheter Removal or Catheter Exchange

Meta-analysis from three studies (499 cases in the coated and 502 cases in the non-coated group) showed no significant risk in the need for catheter removal or exchange (OR 0.93 95% CI 0.52–1.65, p = 0.80) (Figure 4). There was no significant heterogeneity among the studies (I^2 = 0%).

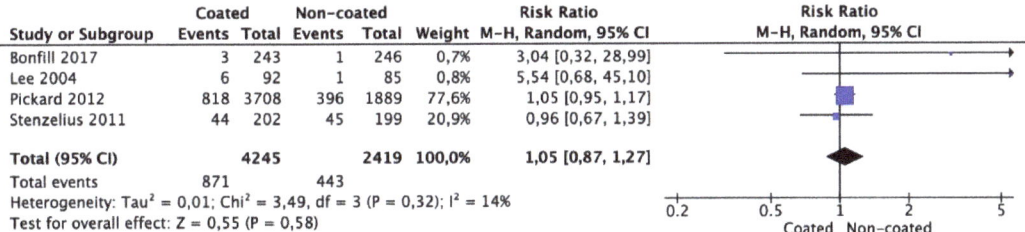

Figure 4. Meta-analysis of need for removal/change of catheter.

3.4. Meta-Analysis of Lower Urinary Tract Symptoms at Follow-Up after Removal of Catheter

Meta-analysis from four studies (4245 cases in the coated and 2419 cases in the non-coated group) showed that the number of patients complaining of lower urinary tract symptoms after catheter removal did not differ between the groups (OR 1.05 95% CI 0.87–1.17, p = 0.58) (Figure 5). There was no significant heterogeneity among the studies (I^2 = 14%).

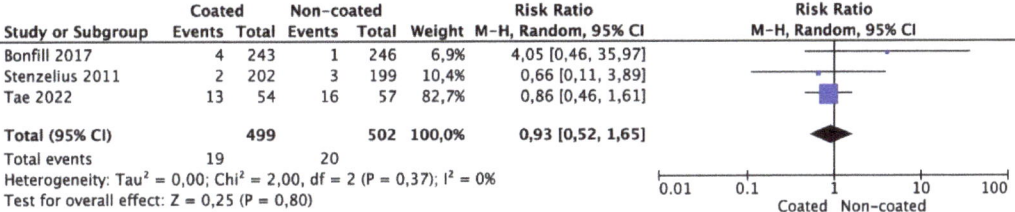

Figure 5. Meta-analysis of the number of patients reporting lower urinary tract symptoms at follow-up after removal of catheter.

3.5. Meta-Analysis of Hematuria Incidence

There was only one study reporting hematuria, making meta-analysis not feasible.

4. Discussion

In our meta-analysis, we found no difference in the incidence of CAUTI in patients with coated and non-coated catheters even though subgroup analysis regarding dwelling time (short- vs. long-term catheterization) showed a significantly lower risk for CAUTI in patients using coated catheters (p = 0.04). The interest in developing catheters that can decrease the risk of CAUTI started in 1979 with Akyama and Okamoto, who were the first to describe a decreased risk for bacteria associated with coated urinary catheters [21]. Other studies reported only a "protective effect" of coated urinary tract catheters but these trials were performed with a small number of patients [19,22,23]. Thibon et al. evaluated the effects of coated catheters with hydrogel and silver salts on the incidence of hospital-acquired urinary tract infection and showed no protective effect of coated catheters [19]. With regard to studies that reported a significant reduction in CAUTI in patients on silver-alloy catheters [12,22,23], some methodological critiques were made to these studies as they were performed by randomizing the hospital unit instead of the individual patients, which could lead to bias since hospital units can differ significantly in terms of catheter placement technique, indwelling time, and patient comorbidities.

Another confounding factor in considering indwelling catheters and CAUTI risk is the surgical procedure performed. Ideally, catheters should be removed at the earliest possible time. The misconception that the use of antibiotic- or silver-coated catheters has better outcomes in patients undergoing urological procedures needing a short duration of catheterization was refuted in a study by Pickard et al. [7]. Likewise, Erickson et al. compared silicone- and hydrogel-coated latex catheters in men needing short-term postoperative bladder drainage after urethral surgeries and showed no absolute advantage for either type [16]. Menzies et al. compared nitrofurazone-coated and non-coated urinary catheters in kidney transplant recipients and did not find any difference in the rate of urinary tract infection (8% and 6.8%, $p = 0.99$) among the two groups [11]. Instead, the incidence of adverse events was more frequent in the nitrofurazone-impregnated silicone urinary catheter group (46.6% and 26.1%, $p = 0.007$) [11]. Tae et al. studied the incidence of CAUTI in patients who underwent radical cystectomy with an orthotopic neobladder for bladder cancer and received either a coated or conventional non-coated catheter for 2 weeks [20]. The incidence of CAUTI 2 weeks after radical cystectomy and orthotopic neobladder was 21.95% (case) and 27.27% (control), with no significant difference between the two groups. However, asymptomatic bacteriuria was significantly lower in the antibiotic-coated catheter group [20]. The authors concluded that the prevention of biofilm formation on coated catheters has the potential to prevent CAUTI. One explanation for why the CAUTI rate was similar between the groups is that the duration of catheterization was short for this cohort (2 weeks); as we demonstrated in our meta-analysis, coated catheters may only be of benefit during longer catheterization durations. When taken together, the results of the present meta-analysis (Figure 3) support the safety of using non-coated catheters in patients undergoing surgical procedures in which catheter duration is expected to be less than 14 days. For patients requiring long-term catheters, the use of coated catheters may lower the risk of CAUTI together with routine catheter and/or drainage bag changes [24].

In a randomized trial of 17 patients, Priefer et al. observed that the practice of monthly catheter exchange resulted in fewer symptomatic urinary tract infections when compared to patients in whom catheters were exchanged at the time of either obstruction or infection [25]. In contrast, White et al. found that when patients were divided into short- versus long-term catheter exchange intervals, the incidence of infection was greater in those whose catheters were changed in 2 weeks or less [26]. Only 15.4% remained free of infection after one month in this group, whereas 80% of those whose catheters were changed between 4 and 6 weeks remained free of infection after 6 weeks. The number of exchange and the number of nurses who performed the catheter exchange might have influenced the CAUTI risk. Indeed, there is insufficient evidence to assess the value of different policies for replacing long-term urinary catheters on patient outcomes [24]. We found that the incidence of CAUTI was decreased when maintained well even for a long duration (RR 0.82 95% CI 0.68–0.99, $p = 0.04$). Thus, maybe the implementation of protocols using coated catheters could be of interest to prevent encrustation, obstruction, and infection, and increase the intervals between changes.

Adverse events related to catheter use, such as hematuria, irritative lower urinary tract symptoms, or the need for catheter exchange or removal, were investigated as secondary endpoints in our study. Only one article classified the infections by differentiating into cystitis or urinary sepsis, preventing our analysis from evaluating these secondary outcomes. Furthermore, no studies comparing coated versus non-coated catheters evaluated rates of pyelonephritis. There were insufficient data to determine the relative influence of coated urinary catheters on hematuria. Hematuria, which was reported in only a single study, occurred in 18/243 (7.4%) patients in the silver alloy-coated catheter group and 20/246 (8.1%) patients using conventional catheters and this was not significantly different between groups [18]. Three studies involving a total of 1001 patients reported on the need for catheter removal or exchange. Overall, the need for urinary catheter exchange or removal was similar between non-coated and coated catheters [14,18,20]. In our analysis, four studies, which included 6664 patients, provided information on lower urinary tract symptoms (LUTS) after catheter removal [7,14,17,18]. LUTS ranged from 1.2% to 22% in the coated group and from 0.4% to 22.6% in the control group. Compared to standard urinary catheters, we found that the use of coated catheters did not significantly increase the risk of LUTS.

Salient to the discussion of comparing antibiotic- or alloy-coated catheters to conventional silicone/latex catheters is cost-effectiveness. Overall, four studies incorporate cost-effectiveness analyses [12,27–29]. Cost analyses can be further stratified into comparisons of cost among different catheters and their associated components as well as analyses incorporating both catheter costs as well as the estimated cost of consequent nosocomial urinary tract infections. The latter cost assessment can be challenging to perform as it may be difficult to delineate how much a CAUTI contributes to the length of hospital stay or utilization of hospital resources. Nonetheless, several studies have provided estimates of these costs.

In a 12-month randomized crossover trial comparing CAUTI rates in patients with silver alloy-coated versus non-coated catheters, the use of silver alloy-coated catheters was associated with a 2.5-fold higher direct material cost when compared to non-coated catheters [12]. However, when taking into account the estimated costs associated with CAUTI and associated sequela (i.e., bloodstream infection, upper tract involvement, need for intensive care unit stay) within their study population, the use of silver alloy-coated catheters yielded significant aggregate savings due to a reduction in CAUTI rates. The lower and higher estimate of cost savings were USD 14,000 and 500,000, respectively [12]. This finding was similarly demonstrated by Bologna et al., where the use of silver alloy-coated catheters was predicted to lead to superior cost savings over standard latex catheters [27]. However, this cost analysis was limited to a single institution, whose differential CAUTI rate between silver alloy-coated and standard silicone catheters significantly differed from that of the other four institutions included in the analysis. The authors also relied on estimates of cost savings by attributing CAUTI as a major driver of hospital and intensive care unit length of stay [27]. Importantly, a recent prospective crossover study comparing silver alloy-coated to standard silicone catheters demonstrated a 12% risk reduction against CAUTI with the use of silver alloy-coated catheters. This is contrary to a prior study that assumed a 30–40% relative reduction in the CAUTI rate with the use of silver alloy-coated catheters in their cost-effectiveness analyses [29]. Therefore, if the difference in the CAUTI rate between catheter types is modest, the cost savings with the use of silver alloy-coated catheters may be negated and may not outweigh the increased direct costs associated with these catheters [29].

In another large study involving 7102 patients admitted to NHS England hospitals, cost-effectiveness analysis demonstrated that nitrofurazone-coated catheters were the least costly [30]. When compared to nitrofurazone-coated catheters, PTFE and silver alloy-coated catheters cost on average USD 11 and 19 more, respectively. Based on their analysis, nitrofurazone-coated catheters had an approximately 70% chance of being a cost-saving and had an 84% chance of having an incremental cost per quality-adjusted life year [incremental cost-effectiveness ratio of < GBP 300,000 (USD 47,500), the willingness-to-pay threshold suggested by the UK National Institute of Health and Clinical Excellence] [30]. Conversely, silver alloy-coated catheters had a 0% chance of being cost-effective at all threshold values between GBP 0 and 50,000. Nonetheless, nitrofurazone-coated catheters were associated with greater patient discomfort and the cost-saving estimates were based on assumptions of large attribution of CAUTI as the main driver of the length of hospital stay. These results, therefore, do not provide robust evidence of cost-effectiveness for one catheter over another within a universal health care system [30].

When taken together, the use of metal alloy-coated or antibiotic-coated catheters may increase direct costs to health care systems when compared to standard silicone or latex catheters; however, it is unclear whether the risk reduction in the CAUTI rate (and associated health care utilization) outweighs this cost.

Our study has some limitations. This study precludes us from making absolute deductions on which coated catheters are better for minimizing CAUTI, and better clinical trials should address this in the future. We could deduce that patients with long-term indwelling catheters could be the ideal candidates for coated catheters and it is necessary to provide proper training to patients and caregivers for catheter maintenance. This could help optimize the cost-effectiveness for the patients as, from our results, due to paucity of information and likely variability in health care systems, it was difficult to make concrete conclusions on cost-effectiveness. Finally, there was no randomized clinical trial comparing coated vs. non-coated suprapubic catheters, considering that UTI incidence is not significantly different between urethral and suprapubic catheters in spinal cord injury and neurogenic bladder [31].

5. Conclusions

In this systematic review of randomized trials, we found that the use of indwelling coated catheters was not associated with a lower incidence of CAUTI and the need for removal/change of catheter compared to non-coated catheters. In addition, we also found no difference in lower urinary tract symptoms after catheter removal. However, the incidence of CUATI was significantly lower using silver alloy-coated catheters in patients who require more than 14 days of dwelling time. The utility of coated catheters to reduce CAUTI risk versus standard catheters must be balanced with differences in direct costs to patients and health care systems.

Author Contributions: Conceptualization, V.G., B.K.S. and J.d.l.R.; methodology, V.G. and D.C.; data gathering, V.G., D.C., C.N., G.C., A.T.G., R.D.d.S., F.L.H., J.Y.-C.T. and M.L.W.; validation, B.K.S., J.Y.-C.T., A.B.G. and J.d.l.R.; formal analysis, D.C.; writing—original draft preparation, V.G., D.C., C.N., G.C., A.T.G., R.D.d.S., F.L.H. and M.L.W.; writing—review and editing, D.C., V.G., B.K.S., A.B.G., J.Y.-C.T. and J.d.l.R. All authors have read and agreed to the published version of the manuscript.

Funding: This research received no external funding.

Data Availability Statement: Data will be provide by the corresponding author upon a reasonable request.

Conflicts of Interest: The authors declare no conflict of interest.

References

1. Feneley, R.C.L.; Hopley, I.B.; Wells, P.N.T. Urinary Catheters: History, Current Status, Adverse Events and Research Agenda. *J. Med. Eng. Technol.* **2015**, *39*, 459–470. [CrossRef] [PubMed]
2. Andersen, M.J.; Flores-Mireles, A.L. Urinary Catheter Coating Modifications: The Race against Catheter-Associated Infections. *Coatings* **2020**, *10*, 23. [CrossRef]
3. Henly, E.L.; Dowling, J.A.R.; Maingay, J.B.; Lacey, M.M.; Smith, T.J.; Forbes, S. Biocide Exposure Induces Changes in Susceptibility, Pathogenicity, and Biofilm Formation in Uropathogenic Escherichia Coli. *Antimicrob. Agents Chemother.* **2019**, *63*, e01892-18. [CrossRef]
4. Kazmierska, K.A.; Thompson, R.; Morris, N.; Long, A.; Ciach, T. In Vitro Multicompartmental Bladder Model for Assessing Blockage of Urinary Catheters: Effect of Hydrogel Coating on Dynamics of Proteus Mirabilis Growth. *Urology* **2010**, *76*, 515.e15–515.e20. [CrossRef] [PubMed]
5. Desai, D.G.; Liao, K.S.; Cevallos, M.E.; Trautner, B.W. Silver or Nitrofurazone Impregnation of Urinary Catheters Has a Minimal Effect on Uropathogen Adherence. *J. Urol.* **2010**, *184*, 2565–2571. [CrossRef] [PubMed]
6. Lam, T.B.L.; Omar, M.I.; Fisher, E.; Gillies, K.; MacLennan, S. Types of Indwelling Urethral Catheters for Short-Term Catheterisation in Hospitalised Adults. *Cochrane Database Syst. Rev.* **2014**, *9*, CD004013. [CrossRef] [PubMed]
7. Pickard, R.; Lam, T.; MacLennan, G.; Starr, K.; Kilonzo, M.; McPherson, G.; Gillies, K.; McDonald, A.; Walton, K.; Buckley, B.; et al. Antimicrobial Catheters for Reduction of Symptomatic Urinary Tract Infection in Adults Requiring Short-Term Catheterisation in Hospital: A Multicentre Randomised Controlled Trial. *Lancet* **2012**, *380*, 1927–1935. [CrossRef]
8. Higgins, J.P.; Eldridge, S.; Tianjing, L. How to Include Multiple Groups from One Study. Available online: https://training.cochrane.org/handbook/current/chapter-23#section-23-3 (accessed on 15 May 2022).
9. Higgins, J.P.T.; Altman, D.G.; Gøtzsche, P.C.; Jüni, P.; Moher, D.; Oxman, A.D.; Savovic, J.; Schulz, K.F.; Weeks, L.; Sterne, J.A.C. The Cochrane Collaboration's Tool for Assessing Risk of Bias in Randomised Trials. *BMJ* **2011**, *343*, d5928. [CrossRef] [PubMed]

10. Akcam, F.Z.; Kaya, O.; Temel, E.N.; Buyuktuna, S.A.; Unal, O.; Yurekli, V.A. An Investigation of the Effectiveness against Bacteriuria of Silver-Coated Catheters in Short-Term Urinary Catheter Applications: A Randomized Controlled Study. *J. Infect. Chemother.* **2019**, *25*, 797–800. [CrossRef]
11. Menezes, F.G.; Corrêa, L.; Medina-Pestana, J.O.; Aguiar, W.F.; Camargo, L.F.A. A Randomized Clinical Trial Comparing Nitrofurazone-Coated and Uncoated Urinary Catheters in Kidney Transplant Recipients: Results from a Pilot Study. *Transpl. Infect. Dis.* **2019**, *21*, e13031. [CrossRef] [PubMed]
12. Karchmer, T.B.; Giannetta, E.T.; Muto, C.A.; Strain, B.A.; Farr, B.M. A Randomized Crossover Study of Silver-Coated Urinary Catheters in Hospitalized Patients. *Arch. Intern. Med.* **2000**, *160*, 3294–3298. [CrossRef] [PubMed]
13. Johnson, J.R.; Roberts, P.L.; Olsen, R.J.; Moyer, K.A.; Stamm, W.E. Prevention of Catheter-Associated Urinary Tract Infection with a Silver Oxide-Coated Urinary Catheter: Clinical and Microbiologic Correlates. *J. Infect. Dis.* **1990**, *162*, 1145–1150. [CrossRef] [PubMed]
14. Stenzelius, K.; Persson, S.; Olsson, U.-B.; Stjärneblad, M. Noble Metal Alloy-Coated Latex versus Silicone Foley Catheter in Short-Term Catheterization: A Randomized Controlled Study. *Scand. J. Urol. Nephrol.* **2011**, *45*, 258–264. [CrossRef] [PubMed]
15. Stensballe, J.; Tvede, M.; Looms, D.; Lippert, F.K.; Dahl, B.; Tønnesen, E.; Rasmussen, L.S. Infection Risk with Nitrofurazone-Impregnated Urinary Catheters in Trauma Patients: A Randomized Trial. *Ann. Intern. Med.* **2007**, *147*, 285–293. [CrossRef] [PubMed]
16. Erickson, B.A.; Navai, N.; Patil, M.; Chang, A.; Gonzalez, C.M. A Prospective, Randomized Trial Evaluating the Use of Hydrogel Coated Latex versus All Silicone Urethral Catheters after Urethral Reconstructive Surgery. *J. Urol.* **2008**, *179*, 203–206. [CrossRef] [PubMed]
17. Lee, S.-J.; Kim, S.W.; Cho, Y.-H.; Shin, W.-S.; Lee, S.E.; Kim, C.-S.; Hong, S.J.; Chung, B.H.; Kim, J.J.; Yoon, M.S. A Comparative Multicentre Study on the Incidence of Catheter-Associated Urinary Tract Infection between Nitrofurazone-Coated and Silicone Catheters. *Int. J. Antimicrob. Agents* **2004**, *24* (Suppl. S1), S65–S659. [CrossRef]
18. Bonfill, X.; Rigau, D.; Esteban-Fuertes, M.; Barrera-Chacón, J.M.; Jáuregui-Abrisqueta, M.L.; Salvador, S.; Alemán-Sánchez, C.M.; Borau, A.; Bea-Muñoz, M.; Hidalgo, B.; et al. Efficacy and Safety of Urinary Catheters with Silver Alloy Coating in Patients with Spinal Cord Injury: A Multicentric Pragmatic Randomized Controlled Trial. The ESCALE Trial. *Spine J.* **2017**, *17*, 1650–1657. [CrossRef]
19. Thibon, P.; Le Coutour, X.; Leroyer, R.; Fabry, J. Randomized Multi-Centre Trial of the Effects of a Catheter Coated with Hydrogel and Silver Salts on the Incidence of Hospital-Acquired Urinary Tract Infections. *J. Hosp. Infect.* **2000**, *45*, 117–124. [CrossRef]
20. Tae, B.S.; Oh, J.J.; Jeong, B.C.; Ku, J.H. Catheter-Associated Urinary Tract Infections in Patients Who Have Undergone Radical Cystectomy for Bladder Cancer: A Prospective Randomized Clinical Study of Two Silicone Catheters (Clinical Benefit of Antibiotic Silicone Material). *Investig. Clin. Urol.* **2022**, *63*, 334–340. [CrossRef] [PubMed]
21. Akiyama, H.; Okamoto, S. Prophylaxis of Indwelling Urethral Catheter Infection: Clinical Experience with a Modified Foley Catheter and Drainage System. *J. Urol.* **1979**, *121*, 40–42. [CrossRef]
22. Liedberg, H.; Lundeberg, T. Silver Alloy Coated Catheters Reduce Catheter-Associated Bacteriuria. *Br. J. Urol.* **1990**, *65*, 379–381. [CrossRef]
23. Liedberg, H.; Lundeberg, T.; Ekman, P. Refinements in the Coating of Urethral Catheters Reduces the Incidence of Catheter-Associated Bacteriuria. An Experimental and Clinical Study. *Eur. Urol.* **1990**, *17*, 236–240. [CrossRef] [PubMed]
24. Cooper, F.P.M.; Alexander, C.E.; Sinha, S.; Omar, M.I. Policies for Replacing Long-Term Indwelling Urinary Catheters in Adults. *Cochrane Database Syst. Rev.* **2016**, *7*, CD011115. [CrossRef] [PubMed]
25. Priefer, B.A.; Duthie, E.H.J.; Gambert, S.R. Frequency of Urinary Catheter Change and Clinical Urinary Tract Infection. Study in Hospital-Based, Skilled Nursing Home. *Urology* **1982**, *20*, 141–142. [CrossRef]
26. White, M.C.; Ragland, K.E. Urinary Catheter-Related Infections among Home Care Patients. *J. Wound Ostomy Cont. Nurs.* **1995**, *22*, 286–290. [CrossRef] [PubMed]
27. Bologna, R.A.; Tu, L.M.; Polansky, M.; Fraimow, H.D.; Gordon, D.A.; Whitmore, K.E. Hydrogel/Silver Ion-Coated Urinary Catheter Reduces Nosocomial Urinary Tract Infection Rates in Intensive Care Unit Patients: A Multicenter Study. *Urology* **1999**, *54*, 982–987. [CrossRef]
28. Chung, P.H.; Wong, C.W.; Lai, C.K.; Siu, H.K.; Tsang, D.N.; Yeung, K.Y.; Ip, D.K.; Tam, P.K. A Prospective Interventional Study to Examine the Effect of a Silver Alloy and Hydrogel-Coated Catheter on the Incidence of Catheter-Associated Urinary Tract Infection. *Hong Kong Med. J.* **2017**, *23*, 239–245. [CrossRef] [PubMed]
29. Srinivasan, A.; Karchmer, T.; Richards, A.; Song, X.; Perl, T.M. A Prospective Trial of a Novel, Silicone-Based, Silver-Coated Foley Catheter for the Prevention of Nosocomial Urinary Tract Infections. *Infect. Control Hosp. Epidemiol.* **2006**, *27*, 38–43. [CrossRef] [PubMed]
30. Pickard, R.; Lam, T.; Maclennan, G.; Starr, K.; Kilonzo, M.; McPherson, G.; Gillies, K.; McDonald, A.; Walton, K.; Buckley, B.; et al. Types of Urethral Catheter for Reducing Symptomatic Urinary Tract Infections in Hospitalised Adults Requiring Short-Term Catheterisation: Multicentre Randomised Controlled Trial and Economic Evaluation of Antimicrobial- and Antiseptic-Impregnated Urethra. *Health Technol. Assess.* **2012**, *16*, 1–197. [CrossRef] [PubMed]
31. Kinnear, N.; Barnett, D.; O'Callaghan, M.; Horsell, K.; Gani, J.; Hennessey, D. The Impact of Catheter-Based Bladder Drainage Method on Urinary Tract Infection Risk in Spinal Cord Injury and Neurogenic Bladder: A Systematic Review. *Neurourol. Urodyn.* **2020**, *39*, 854–862. [CrossRef] [PubMed]

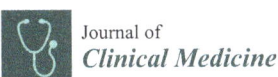

Opinion

Low- vs. High-Power Laser for Holmium Laser Enucleation of Prostate

Vasileios Gkolezakis [1], Bhaskar Kumar Somani [2] and Theodoros Tokas [3,4,*]

1 Department of Urology, Athens Medical Centre, Distomou 5-7, 151 25 Marousi, Greece
2 Department of Urology, University Hospital Southampton NHS Trust, Southampton SO16 6YD, UK
3 Department of Urology and Andrology, General Hospital Hall i.T., Milser Str. 10., A-6060 Hall in Tirol, Austria
4 Training and Research in Urological Surgery and Technology (T.R.U.S.T.)-Group, Milser Str. 10., A-6060 Hall in Tirol, Austria
* Correspondence: ttokas@yahoo.com; Tel.: +43-(0)50-504-36310; Fax: +43-(0)50-504-36313

Abstract: Holmium laser enucleation of the prostate (HoLEP) constitutes an established technique for treating patients with symptomatic bladder outlet obstruction. Most surgeons perform surgeries using high-power (HP) settings. Nevertheless, HP laser machines are costly, require high-power sockets, and may be linked with increased postoperative dysuria. Low-power (LP) lasers could overcome these drawbacks without compromising postoperative outcomes. Nevertheless, there is a paucity of data regarding LP laser settings during HoLEP, as most endourologists are hesitant to apply them in their clinical practice. We aimed to provide an up-to-date narrative looking at the impact of LP settings in HoLEP and comparing LP with HP HoLEP. According to current evidence, intra- and post-operative outcomes as well as complication rates are independent of the laser power level. LP HoLEP is feasible, safe, and effective and may improve postoperative irritative and storage symptoms.

Keywords: prostate enucleation; laser power; holmium; HoLEP

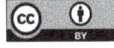

1. Introduction

Benign prostate hyperplasia (BPH) with consecutive lower urinary tract symptoms (LUTS) constitutes a significant health issue of the aging male. Traditional transurethral resection of the prostate (TURP) remains the standard treatment for small- and medium-sized prostate glands and patients who fail medical therapy and may have complications of outlet obstruction such as bladder stones, urinary retention, or renal insufficiency [1]. Nonetheless, between several surgical treatment modalities, transurethral holmium laser enucleation of the prostate (HoLEP) has emerged as a distinctive technique that can be applied to prostates of all sizes [2–4]. Compared to standard TURP, HoLEP offers better hemostasis, shorter catheterization and hospitalization times, and nullifies the rate of TURP syndrome [3,5]. The holmium laser technology enables the prostatic tissue to be enucleated from the capsule while simultaneously coagulating the capsular surface. HoLEP, which offers long-term functional results superior to TURP and comparable to open simple prostatectomy but with lower treatment morbidity and complication rates, is therefore regarded as a procedure of reference for the surgical treatment of large prostate glands [2–4]. Surgeons usually apply power settings of 80–100 W with 2 J energy and 40–50 Hz frequency and an occasional power reduction for coagulation (75 W, 1.5 J, and 50 Hz) and apical preparation (30 W, 0.6 J, and 50 Hz) [6,7]. These settings provide the ability to adjust pulse duration to energy and frequency but also necessitate more expensive equipment with numerous high-power plugs, which are generally considered limitations of the widespread adoption of HoLEP.

Low-power (LP) devices are also available on the market, functioning at powers of 20, 30, and 50 W with lower startup costs and no demand for specialized plugs. The same equipment can be used successfully for lithotripsy and BPH surgery. Comparing these qualities to high-power (HP) units could be advantageous. Rassweiler et al. were the first to use LP settings (24 W, 2 J, and 12 Hz, or 39.6 W, 2.2 J, and 18 Hz) to treat 129 patients, proving the treatment's viability, safety, and effectiveness [7]. These findings implied a significant reduction in the initial capital equipment cost, which may make adopting this technique more bearable if the method's effectiveness is preserved. Despite this, the LP method has not gained much support, and there are still few reports on LP HoLEP in the era of rising HP machine output. On the other hand, the higher price tag that comes with these sophisticated devices is a significant disadvantage, and many endourologists are looking for less expensive options. Furthermore, while HP and unique technologies like MOSES may only be available in referral centers, LP holmium laser machines are universally available, as they are frequently adopted for other endourological procedures (i.e., lithotripsy). Hence, this work aimed to compare LP to standard HP HoLEP regarding perioperative parameters, complications, and functional outcomes.

2. Materials and Methods

2.1. Literature Search

We performed a literature search in PubMed and used the following keywords: 'prostat* hypertrophy', 'prostat* hyperplasia', 'BPH', 'BPO', 'HoLEP', and 'holmium laser'. We limited our search to papers written in English.

2.2. Selection Criteria

The PICOS (patient, intervention, comparison, outcome, study type) model was employed. Patient: adults undergoing HoLEP for BPH; intervention: LP HoLEP; comparison: HP HoLEP; outcome: surgical time, operative efficiency, postoperative catheterization time, length of hospital stay, re-catheterization, blood transfusion, incontinence rate, international prostate symptom score (IPSS), maximum peak flow (Qmax), and post-void residual urine (PVR) at last follow-up; study type: randomized, prospective non-randomized, and retrospective studies. HP HoLEP was conducted at 100 W, whereas LP was performed at 30 W, 40 W, and 50 W. Due to study heterogeneity and the non-standardized quality appraisal, we performed a narrative synthesis. The limitations of using a single database for a review are also taken into account [8]. Furthermore, our results might be constrained by study heterogeneity and selection bias. We included randomized, prospective non-randomized, and retrospective studies and excluded case studies, reviews, and editorials.

3. Results

The literature search identified 969 records (Figure 1). Additionally, we included four studies from other sources. Following title, abstract, and full-text screening, we selected and included 11 studies in the review (Tables 1 and 2). Five studies described the functions and presented outcomes of LP HoLEP and six compared LP with HP HoLEP in terms of procedure times, peri- and postoperative outcomes, and complications. We included four meeting abstracts [9–12], one prospective comparative study [13], one prospective randomized trial [14], one prospective case series [15], three retrospective case series [16–18] and one ex vivo porcine study [19].

3.1. Efficiency and Speed of LP HoLEP

Operative time (OT), enucleation time (ET), operative efficiency (OE; defined as resected prostate weight divided by operative time in g/min), enucleation efficiency (EE; defined as resected prostate weight divided by enucleation time in g/min), laser/prostate ratio (defined as laser energy consumed divided by resected prostate weight, in KJ/g), and laser rate (defined as the laser energy consumed) were among the outcome measures evaluated. In the first randomized controlled trial comparing LP (50 W, 2 J, and 25 Hz) versus traditional HoLEP (100 W, 2 J, and 50 Hz), the authors found comparable outcomes in terms of EE (1.42 ± 0.6 g/min vs. 1.47 ± 0.6 g/min), OE (1.01 ± 0.4 g/min vs. 1.09 ± 0.4 g/min), and OT (81 min vs. 75.5 min) regardless of the surgeon's experience [14].

Two prospective case-control studies from the same group presenting the records of 316 patients with any prostate volume (range 10–200 g), normal PSA, Qmax < 15 mL/s, IPSS > 10, and PVR < 300 cc and comparing the efficacy of en-bloc no-touch LP HoLEP (40 W, 2 J, and 20 Hz) with HP HoLEP (100 W, 2 J, and 50 Hz) revealed identical results regarding mean ET (27.5 min vs. 31 min) and EE (1.7 g/min vs. 1.64 g/min, respectively) in the hands of an experienced surgeon [10,11]. The authors reported a reduction in energy consumption of nearly one-third.

Gazel et al. compared the impact of two different LP settings on enucleation and hemostasis in 160 patients and recorded increased EE (1.2 vs. 0.78 g/min, $p = 0.001$) while administering 37.5 W (1.5 J and 25 Hz) as opposed to 20 W (1 J and 20 Hz) [17]. In addition, the mean enucleation rate (0.64 vs. 0.88%, $p = 0.001$) and laser efficiency (2.07 vs. 2.12 joule/g, $p = 0.003$) were significantly higher with 37.5 W. The enucleation time was significantly shorter (54 vs. 75.5 min, $p = 0.002$). The authors concluded that using 37.5 W, both enucleation and hemostasis could be performed successfully, while using 100 W in the bladder neck shortens the duration of the procedure. Furthermore, in an experimental ex vivo study, Yilmaz et al. demonstrated that the HP–Ho:YAG's efficiency (evaluated by a numerical measurement of the "tissue pocket" created by separating the fascial layers of a porcine belly, measured in cm^2/min) was reduced by 50% in an LP (3 J and 10 Hz) compared to a medium-power (3 J, 25 Hz) laser setting. Additionally, the authors demonstrated more favorable dissection results with HP systems applying high single-pulse energy, short pulses, and medium frequency [19].

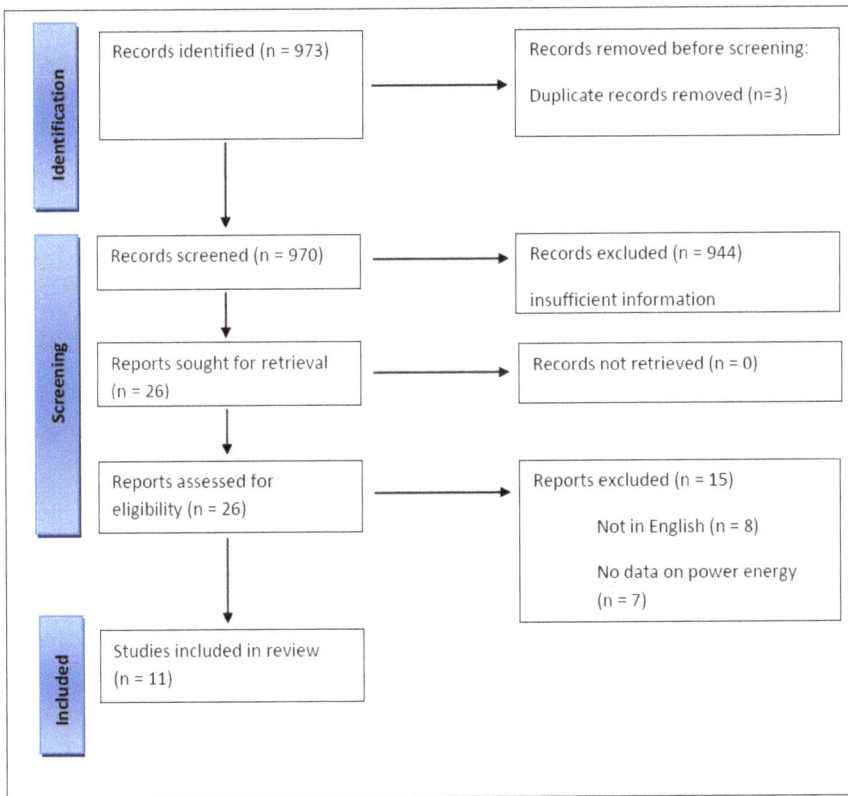

Figure 1. Flow chart.

Table 1. Characteristics of low-power HoLEP studies with initial efficacy parameter.

Author	Design	Laser	Pts (N)	Laser Power	Type of Enucleation	Mean Age ± SD (Years)	Mean PV ± SD (mL)	Mean Adenoma Weight (gr)	Median Time to Catheter Removal (Days) (Range)	Median Hospital Stay (Days)
Becker 2018 [15]	Prospective, not randomized, full text	LP HoLEP	54	2.2 J, 18 Hz~39.6 W	Modified technique	72.5	74.5	46	2	2
Bell 2019 [16]	Retrospective, full text	LP HoLEP (with previous TBP)	24	50 W	3-lobe	66.8 ± 8.2	76.1 ± 35.0	NR	NR	1.3
		LP HoLEP (biopsy-naïve)	85	50 W	3-lobe	71.8 ± 8.7	69.3 ± 31.8	NR	NR	3.0
Gazel 2020 [17]	Retrospective, full text	LP HoLEP	80	1 J, 20 Hz~20 W	3-lobe	63 ± 7.97	79 ± 35.71	NR	42 ± 27.74 (hours)	28 ± 6.06 (hours)
		LP HoLEP	80	1.5 J, 25 Hz~37.5 W	3-lobe	62 ± 7.07	68.5 ± 47.37	NR	27 ± 14.38 (hours)	33 ± 8.03 (hours)
Minagawa 2017 [18]	Retrospective, full text	HP HoLEP	74	1.5 J, 20 Hz~30 W	En-bloc	75.4 ± 7.1	94.5 ± 61.0	51.8	2.6	5.3
Tokatli 2021 [13]	Prospective, randomized, full text	MP HoLEP	60	2.2 J, 18 Hz~39.6 W	2-lobe and 3-lobe	66.5	95	44	2	3
		MP HoLEP	60	1.2 J, 35 Hz~42 W	2-lobe and 3-lobe	67	91	40	2	3

Table 2. Characteristics of included studies comparing low-power vs. high-power holmium laser enucleation of the prostate with initial efficacy parameter.

Author	Design	Laser	Pts (N)	Laser Power	Type of Enucleation	Mean Age ± SD (Years)	Mean PV ± SD (mL)	Mean Adenoma Weight (gr)	Median Time to Catheter Removal (Days) (Range)	Median Hospital Stay (Days)
Gilling 2013 [9]	Prospective, meeting abstract	LP HoLEP HP HoLEP	20 20	50 W 100 W	NR NR	67.4 ± 11.2 68.9 ± 2.0	NR N	22.4 21.7	17.5 (hours) 25.1 (hours)	26.6 (hours) 32.5 (hours)
Scoffone 2017 [10]	Prospective, meeting abstract	LP HoLEP HP HoLEP	102 214	2.2 J, 18 Hz~40 W 2 J, 50 Hz~100 W	En-bloc En-bloc	67.7 ± 8 69.4 ± 7.5	NR NR	46 55	NR NR	NR NR
Cracco 2017 [11]	Prospective, meeting abstract	LP HoLEP HP HoLEP	102 214	2.2 J, 18 Hz~40 W 52 J, 50 Hz~100 W	En-bloc En-bloc	67.7 ± 8 69.4 ± 7.5	NR NR	46 55	NR NR	NR NR
Elshal 2018 [14]	Prospective, randomized controlled trial, full text	LP HoLEP HP HoLEP	61 60	2 J, 25 Hz~50 W 2 J, 50 Hz~100 W	2-lobe and 3-lobe 2-lobe and 3-lobe	66.4 ± 7 67.0 ± 7	137.6 ± 58 137.6 ± 58	75.5 77	1 (1–5) 1 (1–5)	1 (1–3) 1 (1–5)
Cracco 2020 [12]	Retrospective, meeting abstract	LP HoLEP HP HoLEP	326 212	40 W 100 W	Partial and total en-bloc Partial en-bloc	NR NR	NR NR	48,9 53.3	NR NR	NR NR
Yilmaz 2022 [19]	Ex vivo, porcine belly	LP HoLEP HP HoLEP	NR NR	3.5 J, 10 Hz~35 W 4.5 J, 22.2 Hz~100 W	NR NR	NR NR	NR NR	NR NR	NR NR	NR NR

3.2. Functional Outcomes of LP HoLEP

Two prospective studies showed significant improvement in IPSS scores and Qmax at three months (24 vs. 5, $p < 0.001$ and 7.8 mL/s vs. 28 mL/s, $p < 0.001$, respectively) [13] and 12 months follow-up (22 vs. 6, $p < 0.001$ and 12 mL/s vs. 29.3 mL/s, $p < 0.001$, respectively) [14] compared to the preoperative assessment. The authors also observed significant improvements regarding PVR at three months (100 mL vs. 30 mL, $p < 0.001$) and 12 months follow-up (135 mL vs. 11.15 mL, $p < 0.001$) [15]. Gilling et al. prospectively compared LP to HP HoLEP and observed a considerable and persistent improvement in these parameters for both energies at up to 12 months follow-up compared to baseline (30.9 mL/s vs. 7.7 mL/s for 50 W setting, 19 mL/s vs. 7.4 mL/s for 100 W setting, statistical evaluation not reported) [9]. In addition, one prospective comparative study [10] and one randomized trial [14] showed similar results with no difference among LP and HP HoLEP regarding IPSS scores at three months follow-up (6.5 ± 5 d.s. vs. 7.8 ± 5 d.s.) [10] and IPSS scores and Qmax at 12 months follow-up (3 vs. 4, $p = 0.4$, 21.1 mL/s vs. 21.8 mL/s, $p = 0.7$) [14].

3.3. Postoperative Stress Urinary Incontinence (SIU) and Dysuria after LP HoLEP

Becker et al. reported postoperative SIU rates of 16.7% after one month, declining to 0% after six months [15], whereas Gazel et al. showed similar postoperative SIU rates with both 20 W and 37.5 W energy settings (3.7 vs. 2.5% at three months and 1.2 vs. 0% at 12 months follow-up) [17]. Minagawa et al. assessed SIU retrospectively and found that in 55 patients without preoperative SIU, postoperative SIU was observed in seven patients (12.7%) at one month postoperatively and in three patients (5.5%) at three months postoperatively [18]. Scoffone et al. [10] and Elshal et al. [14] demonstrated similar long-lasting incontinence rates at three months (1.6 vs. 1.4%) [10] and four months (1.6 vs. 1.7%) [14] in patients undergoing LP HoLEP and HP HoLEP.

3.4. Safety of LP HoLEP

Reported complication rates of LP HoLEP ranged from 7 to 24% [12]. Of them, 3.7% were Clavien grade 3a, and 5.5% were Clavien 3b [15]. Transfusion rates varied from 0%, with only one case among 74 patients requiring hemostasis under anesthesia (1.3% Clavien grade 3a) [18], to 5% in large adenomas >80 g [12]. The hemoglobin decrease typically varies from 0.5 g/dL [17] to 1.5 g/dL [15]. Tokatli et al. found that patients who had undergone prostate biopsy before HoLEP treatment had a significant hemoglobin drop ($p = 0.002$) regardless of the type of laser device used [13]. The excellent coagulation effect obtained with LP HoLEP was confirmed in the randomized controlled trial by Elshal et al.; the authors found no statistically significant difference between LP and HP HoLEP in median perioperative hemoglobin deficit (0.9 vs. 0.7, $p = 0.6$), blood transfusion rate (0% vs. 0%), median hospital stay (1 day vs. 1 day, $p = 0.052$) and time to catheter removal (1 day vs. 1 day, $p = 0.7$) [14]. Occasionally, LP HoLEP devices produced results that were marginally preferable, such as shorter median catheter times (17.5 vs. 25.1 h) and recovery times (26.6 vs. 32.5 h), although statistical significance was not reached in these cases [9]. When comparing the mean catheterization time (42 h for the 20 W setting vs. 27 h for the 37.5 W setting, $p = 0.008$), Gazel et al. recorded a significant improvement with 37.5 W, whereas no significant difference was found in terms of mean hospitalization time (28 vs. 33 h, $p = 0.16$) [17]. Furthermore, in two prospective and one retrospective LP case series, the median time to catheter removal was 2 [13,15] and 2.6 days [18]. The median hospital stay ranged from 2 [15] to 5.3 days [18]. A statistically significant shorter length of stay was observed in patients with a previous transperineal biopsy (1.3 vs. 3 days, $p < 0.001$) [16].

4. Opinion

Since the initial groundbreaking research [20,21], the HoLEP treatment has advanced alongside other developments in urological technology [2–4]. According to the most recent research, one pedal should deliver a high laser intensity (>80 W) throughout the entire procedure [18,22,23]. While a quick enucleation can be achieved this way, irritative symptoms frequently remain even a year later [18]. In a recent editorial, Scoffone et al. [23] reported that they retained enucleation effectiveness and efficiency while reducing the laser photothermic effect on the capsule by decreasing the power output from 50 to 20 W. Several authors backed this finding by showing that LP is just as effective as HP HoLEP [12,15,18]. Cecchetti et al.'s "in-vitro" research [24] convincingly showed how different holmium laser settings interact with shockwaves and produce temperatures on soft tissues. The researchers demonstrated that the lowest threshold for plasma bubble generation and shockwave noise for soft tissue ablation was detected at an energy level of 1.4 J and a frequency of 10 Hz. With a particular quantity of joules provided at a lower frequency and an additional longer pulse duration, thermal relaxation time is significantly increased, fewer photothermic side effects are created, and the photomechanical effects are softened while also maintaining laser effectiveness [24,25]. However, it is crucial to remember that while the frequency can be dropped somewhat proportionately, the energy should not be decreased significantly [26].

It is challenging to predict how a laser will affect a particular type of tissue because of the complex interactions between the laser (wavelength, absorption coefficient, power, and pulse), tissue (water concentration, hardness, and absorption coefficient), environment (air and liquid), and the distance and inclination angle between the fibre tip and tissue [27]. A vaporization zone (vaporization volume), incision depth, width, coagulation zone, carbonization zone, and thermo-mechanical or laser damage zone are the parameters that define laser incisions, which are created by explosive tissue water vaporization [28]. Protein denaturation and pyrolysis induce thermal coagulation to develop between 60 and 100 °C. The release of carbon atoms after the vaporization of water molecules causes the adjacent tissue to become carbonized [29]. Perfusion simplifies the process of transferring heat from the laser incision into healthy tissue below, reducing heat damage. However, perfused and non-perfused porcine kidneys show similar laser damage zones [30]. The type of laser used during endoscopic prostate enucleation can affect the type of incision and the power settings used [31]. Using HP lasers, faster procedure times and more significant hemostasis can be achieved, along with broader and deeper tissue incisions [32]. However, when operating near the prostate pseudo-capsule, deeper incisions, especially with a more expansive thermo-mechanical damage zone, may result in collateral damage, such as a neurovascular bundle injury [4]. In contrast, the minimal carbonization zone associated with LP lasers might reduce postoperative urge symptoms [33] and improve histological findings [28].

The most crucial distinction between LP and HP HoLEP is operational effectiveness. The primary evidence for the efficiency of LP HoLEP was provided by the single-series retrospective investigation by Minagawa et al. [18]. In this study, HoLEP procedures were carried out using an 80 W device with a 30 W power setting by surgeons with various surgical skills. HoLEP was successfully treated on every occasion, regardless of the LP setting, without increasing the laser's output, and no patient required a blood transfusion. Furthermore, the authors assessed the outcomes while considering the surgeon's level of expertise and concluded that the enucleation time was significantly reduced when an experienced surgeon carried out the HoLEP operation. Moreover, the EE results aligned with other publications that used an HP laser.

The level of surgical experience may be a significant confounder affecting the procedure results. Without utilizing a control group, a study looked at the EE of HoLEP surgery performed by two experienced surgeons using a 50 W device (2.2 J and 18 Hz) [15]. The authors found that their EE values were higher than those reached by HP laser devices after comparing their results to those of earlier HP HoLEP series. They also stressed that the surgeon's experience is more crucial than the device's power for acquiring high EE values. Elshal et al. [14] observed no statistically significant differences between the two groups for any operational parameters, including EE values, in the first randomized controlled experiment contrasting LP HoLEP vs. conventional HP HoLEP (50 W and 100 W energy settings). When contrasting the findings of studies comparing the effects of various energy settings on the efficiency of enucleation during the HoLEP procedure, it is apparent that EE values were reported to be lower in studies conducted before 2013 (mean EE values ranged between 0.45 and 0.94 g/min) [7,34] compared with studies conducted in 2017 or later (mean EE values ranged between 1.1 and 1.7 g/min) [14,15]. These findings demonstrate the importance of gaining experience over time by showing that regardless of the device's power, the procedure's effectiveness improves as the surgeon's experience increases. This conclusion implies that starting HoLEP with large-volume prostates is not advisable for novice surgeons.

Endourologists commonly base their selections on the safety of the procedure and the potential for excessive intraoperative bleeding when selecting the laser settings for HoLEP. Using 25 W vs. 40 W power settings in the initial experiment, Rassweiler et al. [7] discovered an average hemoglobin reduction of 3.1 g/dL and an 8% transfusion rate in their patient groups. Despite the unexpectedly high results, several papers with patients receiving procedures with LP settings have reported acceptable values. In their prospective investigation, Becker et al. [15] used the 39.6 W energy setting on 50 W Ho:YAG laser equipment for HoLEP surgery and collected data on more than 50 patients. They noted a 1.9% transfusion rate and an average hemoglobin decrease of 1.5 g/dL. In a different study comparing 50 W and 100 W energy settings, the decrease in hemoglobin was 0.9 and 0.7 g/dL, respectively [18]. Results from a multiple regression analysis by Tokatli et al. [13] revealed that the sole independent predictor of hemoglobin decline was the existence of biopsy anamnesis. Some underlying factors for the increased bleeding risk include acute or chronic inflammatory reactions that cause granulation in the tissue. HoLEP and removing the adenomatous tissue from the prostatic capsule may also be more challenging to accomplish if there is an inflammatory reaction following the biopsy.

One of the problematic consequences of the HoLEP procedure is postoperative SIU, which can occur to an extent in between 2–15% of patients [35–37]. SIU is typically described as temporary, which is reassuring the patients and adds significantly to the preoperative counseling process [38]. The two leading causes of SIU are significant urethral sphincter traction during surgery and tissue damage caused by laser energy close to the prostate's apex. The likelihood of SIU can be decreased by the adenoma's low energy consumption close to the urethral sphincter. Prospectively, Becker et al. [15] found that the postoperative immediate SIU rate at 1-month follow-up was high (16.7%). However, the rate of SIU decreased to zero by the 6-month follow-up, in line with what is seen with other HP HoLEP series, TURP, and open prostatectomy [3,36,39–41].

Research teams using LP HoLEP report results equivalent to those seen when using HP settings. However, the fact that every surgeon who reports on LP HoLEP uses a different enucleation technique, adding the advantages of each to the LP settings, may be a source of bias. We could also converse concerning how to interpret each outcome measure. For example, the length of stay in the hospital is another indirect indicator that may be highly "environment-dependent" since a surgeon may be reluctant to remove the catheter too soon for fear that doing so will result in an immediate re-catheterization (e.g., hospital stay time is longer in Japan for this reason due to the insurance system). Even enucleation efficiency, which seems to be a very reliable indicator of the intraoperative outcome and reflects both the efficiency of the laser and the clarity of vision in a particular setting, may be influenced by several factors, such as the size of the adenoma (large adenomas significantly improve it, while smaller ones worsen it), so the range of adenoma volume within a case series may influence this factor. Also, the narrative structure of this work underscores the paucity of reliable evidence on this subject. The works included in this study are heterogeneous, particularly regarding the types of laser fibres and the laser and irrigation settings used. In addition, the descriptions of tissue effects during laser ablation differ between study groups in terms of definitions, units, and extra details like laser activation/deactivation intervals or laser tip/tissue distance. The critical endpoints and objectives of the included papers also vary. Further multicentric studies are needed to determine how variables deemed necessary for enucleation, such as prostate size, surgical technique, and surgeon expertise, may alter the outcomes of problems when different holmium machines are used [42].

5. Conclusions

LP HoLEP is feasible, safe, and effective and may help lessen the frequency, severity, and duration of postoperative dysuria and storage symptoms. The laser power level does not significantly affect the intra- and postoperative variables and the complication rates. While more comparative studies are still required to confirm the efficacy of LP HoLEP with various enucleation techniques, the physical background for LP HoLEP is valid and supports its use, encouraging surgeons with access to LP machines to use this method.

Author Contributions: Concept and Study design: T.T.; Methods and experimental work: V.G. and T.T.; Results analysis and conclusions: V.G.; Manuscript preparation: V.G., B.K.S. and T.T. All authors have read and agreed to the published version of the manuscript.

Funding: This research received no external funding.

Institutional Review Board Statement: Not applicable.

Informed Consent Statement: Not applicable.

Data Availability Statement: Not applicable.

Conflicts of Interest: The authors declare no conflict of interest.

References

1. Gratzke, C.; Bachmann, A.; Descazeaud, A.; Drake, M.J.; Madersbacher, S.; Mamoulakis, C.; Oelke, M.; Tikkinen, K.A.; Gravas, S. EAU Guidelines on the Assessment of Non-neurogenic Male Lower Urinary Tract Symptoms including Benign Prostatic Obstruction. *Eur. Urol.* **2015**, *67*, 1099–1109. [CrossRef] [PubMed]
2. Vincent, M.W.; Gilling, P.J. HoLEP has come of age. *World J. Urol.* **2015**, *33*, 487–493. [CrossRef] [PubMed]
3. Cornu, J.-N.; Ahyai, S.; Bachmann, A.; de la Rosette, J.; Gilling, P.; Gratzke, C.; McVary, K.; Novara, G.; Woo, H.; Madersbacher, S. A Systematic Review and Meta-analysis of Functional Outcomes and Complications Following Transurethral Procedures for Lower Urinary Tract Symptoms Resulting from Benign Prostatic Obstruction: An Update. *Eur. Urol.* **2015**, *67*, 1066–1096. [CrossRef] [PubMed]
4. Herrmann, T.R.W.; Liatsikos, E.N.; Nagele, U.; Traxer, O.; Merseburger, A.S. EAU Guidelines on Laser Technologies. *Eur. Urol.* **2012**, *61*, 783–795. [CrossRef]
5. Suardi, N.; Gallina, A.; Salonia, A.; Briganti, A.; Dehò, F.; Zanni, G.; Abdollah, F.; Naspro, R.; Cestari, A.; Guazzoni, G.; et al. Holmium laser enucleation of the prostate and holmium laser ablation of the prostate: Indications and outcome. *Curr. Opin. Urol.* **2009**, *19*, 38–43. [CrossRef]
6. Gong, Y.-G.; He, D.-L.; Wang, M.-Z.; Li, X.-D.; Zhu, G.-D.; Zheng, Z.-H.; Du, Y.-F.; Chang, L.S.; Nan, X.-Y. Holmium Laser Enucleation of the Prostate: A Modified Enucleation Technique and Initial Results. *J. Urol.* **2012**, *187*, 1336–1340. [CrossRef] [PubMed]
7. Rassweiler, J.; Roder, M.; Schulze, M.; Muschter, R. Transurethral enucleation of the prostate with the holmium: YAG laser system: How much power is necessary? *Urologe A* **2008**, *47*, 441–448. [CrossRef]
8. Falagas, M.E.; Pitsouni, E.I.; Malietzis, G.A.; Pappas, G. Comparison of PubMed, Scopus, Web of Science, and Google Scholar: Strengths and weaknesses. *FASEB J.* **2008**, *22*, 338–342. [CrossRef]
9. Gilling, P.; Mason, C.; Reuther, R.; Van Rij, S.; Fraundorfer, M. Use of low-powered HoLEP for the treatment of benign prostatic hyperplasia. *BJU Int.* **2013**, *111* (Suppl. 1), 13–126.
10. Scoffone, C.M.; Ingrosso, M.; Russo, N.; Cracco, C. MP02-10 Low-Power versus High-Power En-Bloc No-Touch Holep: Comparing Feasibility, Safety and Efficacy. *J. Urol.* **2017**, *197* (Suppl. 4), e14. [CrossRef]
11. Cracco, C.; Ingrosso, M.; Russo, N.; Scoffone, C.M. MP02-11 Postoperative Dysuria after High- and Low-Power en-Bloc No-Touch Holep. *J. Urol.* **2017**, *197* (Suppl. 4), e487–e488. [CrossRef]
12. Cracco, C.; Cattaneo, G.; Sica, A.; Ndrevataj, D.; Scoffone, C.M. MP32-08 Impact of Adenoma Volume on the Intraoperative Features of 3 Newly Developed Approaches for Holmium Laser Enucleation of the Prostate. *J. Urol.* **2020**, *203* (Suppl. 4), e487–e488. [CrossRef]
13. Tokatli, Z.; Ferhat, M.; Ibis, M.A.; Sariyildiz, G.T.; Elhan, A.; Sarica, K. Does the power of the laser devices matter for a successful HoLEP procedure? A prospective comparative study. *Int. J. Clin. Pract.* **2021**, *75*, e14531. [CrossRef] [PubMed]
14. Elshal, A.M.; El-Nahas, A.R.; Ghazy, M.; Nabeeh, H.; Laymon, M.; Soltan, M.; Ghobrial, F.K.; El-Kappany, H.A. Low-Power vs. High-Power Holmium Laser Enucleation of the Prostate: Critical Assessment through Randomized Trial. *Urology* **2018**, *121*, 58–65. [CrossRef]

15. Becker, B.; Gross, A.J.; Netsch, C. Safety and efficacy using a low-powered holmium laser for enucleation of the prostate (HoLEP): 12-month results from a prospective low-power HoLEP series. *World J. Urol.* **2018**, *36*, 441–447. [CrossRef] [PubMed]
16. Bell, C.; Moore, S.L.; Gill, A.; Obi-Njoku, O.; Hughes, S.F.; Saleemi, A.; Ellis, G.; Khan, F.; Shergill, I.S. Safety and efficacy of Holmium laser enucleation of the prostate (HoLEP) in patients with previous transperineal biopsy (TPB): Outcomes from a dual-centre case-control study. *BMC Urol.* **2019**, *19*, 97. [CrossRef]
17. Gazel, E.; Kaya, E.; Yalçın, S.; Okas, T.; Aybal, H.C.; Yılmaz, S.; Tunc, L. The low power effect on holmium laser enucleation of prostate (HoLEP): A comparison between 20 W and 37,5 W energy regarding apical enucleation efficacy and patient safety. *Prog. Urol.* **2020**, *30*, 632–638. [CrossRef]
18. Minagawa, S.; Okada, S.; Morikawa, H. Safety and Effectiveness of Holmium Laser Enucleation of the Prostate Using a Low-power Laser. *Urology* **2017**, *110*, 51–55. [CrossRef]
19. Yilmaz, M.; Esser, J.; Kraft, L.; Petzold, R.; Sigle, A.; Gratzke, C.; Suarez-Ibarrola, R.; Miernik, A. Experimental ex-vivo performance study comparing a novel, pulsed thulium solid-state laser, chopped thulium fibre laser, low and high-power holmium:YAG laser for endoscopic enucleation of the prostate. *World J. Urol.* **2022**, *40*, 601–606. [CrossRef]
20. Fraundorfer, M.R.; Gilling, P.J. Holmium:YAG Laser Enucleation of the Prostate Combined with Mechanical Morcellation: Preliminary Results. *Eur. Urol.* **1998**, *33*, 69–72. [CrossRef]
21. Gilling, P.J.; Kennett, K.; Das, A.K.; Thompson, D.; Fraundorfer, M.R. Holmium Laser Enucleation of the Prostate (HoLEP) Combined with Transurethral Tissue Morcellation: An Update on the Early Clinical Experience. *J. Endourol.* **1998**, *12*, 457–459. [CrossRef] [PubMed]
22. Baazeem, A.S.; Elmansy, H.M.; Elhilali, M.M. Holmium Laser Enucleation of the Prostate: Modified Technical Aspects. *BJU Int.* **2010**, *105*, 584–585. [CrossRef] [PubMed]
23. Gilling, P.J.; Aho, T.F.; Frampton, C.M.; King, C.J.; Fraundorfer, M.R. Holmium Laser Enucleation of the Prostate: Results at 6 Years. *Eur. Urol.* **2008**, *53*, 744–749. [CrossRef] [PubMed]
24. Cecchetti, W.; Zattoni, F.; Nigro, F.; Tasca, A. Plasma bubble formation induced by holmium laser: An in vitro study. *Urology* **2004**, *63*, 586–590. [CrossRef] [PubMed]
25. Scoffone, C.M.; Cracco, C.M. High-Power HoLEP: No Thanks! *World J. Urol.* **2018**, *36*, 837–838. [CrossRef]
26. Hardy, L.A.; Kennedy, J.D.; Wilson, C.R.; Irby, P.B.; Fried, N.M. Analysis of thulium fiber laser induced bubble dynamics for ablation of kidney stones. *J. Biophotonics* **2016**, *10*, 1240–1249. [CrossRef]
27. Verdaasdonk, R.; Van Swol, C.F.P.; Grimbergen, M.C.M.; Rem, A.I. Imaging techniques for research and education of thermal and mechanical interactions of lasers with biological and model tissues. *J. Biomed. Opt.* **2006**, *11*, 041110. [CrossRef]
28. Becker, B.; Enikeev, D.; Glybochko, P.; Rapoport, L.; Taratkin, M.; Gross, A.J.; Vinnichenko, V.; Herrmann, T.R.W.; Netsch, C. Effect of optical fiber diameter and laser emission mode (cw vs. pulse) on tissue damage profile using 1.94 μm Tm:fiber lasers in a porcine kidney model. *World J. Urol.* **2019**, *38*, 1563–1568. [CrossRef]
29. Doizi, S.; Germain, T.; Panthier, F.; Compérat, E.; Traxer, O.; Berthe, L. Comparison of Holmium:YAG and Thulium Fiber Lasers on Soft Tissue: An Ex Vivo Study. *J. Endourol.* **2022**, *36*, 251–258. [CrossRef]
30. Khoder, W.Y.; Zilinberg, K.; Waidelich, R.; Stief, C.G.; Becker, A.J.; Pangratz, T.; Hennig, G.; Sroka, R. Ex vivo comparison of the tissue effects of six laser wavelengths for potential use in laser supported partial nephrectomy. *J. Biomed. Opt.* **2012**, *17*, 068005. [CrossRef]
31. Ortner, G.; Rice, P.; Nagele, U.; Herrmann, T.R.W.; Somani, B.K.; Tokas, T. Tissue thermal effect during lithotripsy and tissue ablation in endourology: A systematic review of experimental studies comparing Holmium and Thulium lasers. *World J. Urol.* **2023**, *41*, 1–12. [CrossRef]
32. Enikeev, D.; Glybochko, P.; Rapoport, L.; Okhunov, Z.; O'Leary, M.; Potoldykova, N.; Sukhanov, R.; Enikeev, M.; Laukhtina, E.; Taratkin, M. Impact of endoscopic enucleation of the prostate with thulium fiber laser on the erectile function. *BMC Urol.* **2018**, *18*, 87. [CrossRef] [PubMed]
33. Chen, C.-H.; Chiang, P.-H.; Lee, W.-C.; Chuang, Y.-C.; Kang, C.-H.; Hsu, C.-C.; Chen, Y.-T.; Cheng, Y.-T. High-intensity diode laser in combination with bipolar transurethral resection of the prostate: A new strategy for the treatment of large prostates (>80 mL). *Lasers Surg. Med.* **2012**, *44*, 699–704. [CrossRef] [PubMed]
34. Wisenbaugh, E.S.; Nunez-Nateras, R.; Mmeje, C.O.; Warner, J.N.; Humphreys, M.R. Does prostate morphology affect outcomes after holmium laser enucleation? *Urology* **2013**, *81*, 844–848. [CrossRef] [PubMed]
35. Hurle, R.; Vavassori, I.; Piccinelli, A.; Manzetti, A.; Valenti, S.; Vismara, A. Holmium laser enucleation of the prostate combined with mechanical morcellation in 155 patients with benign prostatic hyperplasia. *Urology* **2002**, *60*, 449–453. [CrossRef]
36. Naspro, R.; Suardi, N.; Salonia, A.; Scattoni, V.; Guazzoni, G.; Colombo, R.; Cestari, A.; Briganti, A.; Mazzoccoli, B.; Rigatti, P.; et al. Holmium Laser Enucleation of the Prostate versus Open Prostatectomy for Prostates >70g: 24-Month Follow-up. *Eur. Urol.* **2006**, *50*, 563–568. [CrossRef]
37. Tan, A.H.; Gilling, P.; Kennett, K.; Frampton, C.; Westenberg, A.; Fraundorfer, M. A Randomized Trial Comparing Holmium Laser Enucleation of the Prostate with Transurethral Resection of the Prostate for the Treatment of Bladder Outlet Obstruction Secondary to Benign Prostatic Hyperplasia in Large Glands (40 to 200 Grams). *J. Urol.* **2003**, *170 Pt 1*, 1270–1274. [CrossRef]
38. Wei, Y.; Ke, Z.; Xu, N.; Xue, X. Complications of anatomical endoscopic enucleation of the prostate. *Andrologia* **2020**, *52*, e13557. [CrossRef]

39. Ahyai, S.A.; Gilling, P.; Kaplan, S.A.; Kuntz, R.M.; Madersbacher, S.; Montorsi, F.; Speakman, M.J.; Stief, C.G. Meta-analysis of Functional Outcomes and Complications Following Transurethral Procedures for Lower Urinary Tract Symptoms Resulting from Benign Prostatic Enlargement. *Eur. Urol.* **2010**, *58*, 384–397. [CrossRef]
40. Gilling, P.J.; Wilson, L.C.; King, C.J.; Westenberg, A.M.; Frampton, C.M.; Fraundorfer, M.R. Long-term results of a randomized trial comparing holmium laser enucleation of the prostate and transurethral resection of the prostate: Results at 7 years. *BJU Int.* **2012**, *109*, 408–411. [CrossRef]
41. Kuntz, R.M.; Lehrich, K.; Ahyai, S.A. Holmium Laser Enucleation of the Prostate versus Open Prostatectomy for Prostates Greater than 100 Grams: 5-Year Follow-Up Results of a Randomised Clinical Trial. *Eur. Urol.* **2008**, *53*, 160–168. [CrossRef] [PubMed]
42. Elzayat, E.; Habib, E.; Elhilali, M. Holmium laser enucleation of the prostate (HoLEP): A size independent new gold standard. *Urology* **2005**, *66* (Suppl. 5), 108–113. [CrossRef] [PubMed]

Disclaimer/Publisher's Note: The statements, opinions and data contained in all publications are solely those of the individual author(s) and contributor(s) and not of MDPI and/or the editor(s). MDPI and/or the editor(s) disclaim responsibility for any injury to people or property resulting from any ideas, methods, instructions or products referred to in the content.

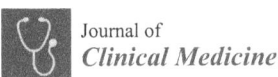

Systematic Review

Radiomics in Urolithiasis: Systematic Review of Current Applications, Limitations, and Future Directions

Ee Jean Lim [1,*], Daniele Castellani [2], Wei Zheng So [3], Khi Yung Fong [3], Jing Qiu Li [1], Ho Yee Tiong [4], Nariman Gadzhiev [5], Chin Tiong Heng [6], Jeremy Yuen-Chun Teoh [7], Nithesh Naik [8], Khurshid Ghani [9], Kemal Sarica [10], Jean De La Rosette [11], Bhaskar Somani [12] and Vineet Gauhar [6]

1 Department of Urology, Singapore General Hospital, Singapore 169608, Singapore
2 Urology Unit, Azienda Ospedaliero-Universitaria Ospedali Riuniti di Ancona, Università Politecnica Delle Marche, 60126 Ancona, Italy
3 Yong Loo Lin School of Medicine, National University of Singapore, Singapore 119077, Singapore
4 Department of Urology, National University Hospital, Singapore 119074, Singapore
5 Department of Urology, Saint-Petersburg State University Hospital, 199034 St. Petersburg, Russia
6 Department of Urology, Ng Teng Fong Hospital, Singapore 609606, Singapore
7 S.H. Ho Urology Centre, Department of Surgery, The Chinese University of Hong Kong, Hong Kong SAR, China
8 Department of Mechanical and Industrial Engineering, Manipal Institute of Technology, Manipal Academy of Higher Education, Manipal 576104, Karnataka, India
9 Department of Urology, University of Michigan, Ann Arbor, MI 48109, USA
10 Department of Urology, Biruni University, 34010 Istanbul, Turkey
11 Istanbul Medipol University, TEM Avrupa Otoyolu Goztepe Cikisi No:1, 34010 Istanbul, Turkey
12 Department of Urology, University Hospital Southampton NHS Foundation Trust, Southampton SO16 6YD, UK
* Correspondence: eejeanlim@gmail.com; Tel.: +65-6321-4693

Abstract: Radiomics is increasingly applied to the diagnosis, management, and outcome prediction of various urological conditions. Urolithiasis is a common benign condition with a high incidence and recurrence rate. The purpose of this scoping review is to evaluate the current evidence of the application of radiomics in urolithiasis, especially its utility in diagnostics and therapeutics. An electronic literature search on radiomics in the setting of urolithiasis was conducted on PubMed, EMBASE, and Scopus from inception to 21 March 2022. A total of 7 studies were included. Radiomics has been successfully applied in the field of urolithiasis to differentiate phleboliths from calculi and classify stone types and composition pre-operatively. More importantly, it has also been utilized to predict outcomes and complications after endourological procedures. Although radiomics in urolithiasis is still in its infancy, it has the potential for large-scale implementation. Its greatest potential lies in the correlation with conventional established diagnostic and therapeutic factors.

Keywords: radiomics; urolithiasis; therapeutic applications

1. Introduction

The exponential growth of medical digitalization and data acquisition has led to the healthcare sector embracing artificial intelligence (AI) to manage and optimize data accruement and utilization [1]. The scope of analysis has correspondingly broadened and introduced a new scientific field collectively called "omics" [2]. The branches of science known informally as omics refers to a field of study in biological sciences that ends with -omics, such as genomics, transcriptomics, proteomics, or metabolomics. The application of AI capabilities within the context of medical imaging is known as radiomics. Radiomics is a quantitative method that primarily extracts extensive amounts of mineable data from medical imaging and radiographic images [3]. These features are subsequently input into statistical frameworks and evaluated. It quantifies textural information by using analysis

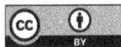

methods from the field of artificial intelligence to analyse "big data" [4]. Big data is defined as "a term that describes large volumes of high velocity, complex and variable data that require advanced techniques and technologies to enable the capture, storage, distribution, management, and analysis of the information" [5]. AI is used for mathematical extraction of the spatial distribution of signal intensities and pixel interrelationships and quantifies textural information which is otherwise imperceptible to humans [6,7]. Radiomics aims at improving precision medicine by using AI to improve diagnostic and prognostic information [8,9]. It surpasses the human ability to identify key imaging characteristics imperceptible to the naked human eye, picking up hidden objective data that may influence subsequent treatment decisions [10].

Data-characterization algorithms such as machine learning (ML), deep learning (DL), and artificial neural networks (ANNs) have already been incorporated to generate radiomics-guided learning models that guide diagnosis, stratification, and treatment [11,12]. In recent years, radiomics has been increasingly applied to the diagnosis, management, and outcome prediction of several medical and urological conditions.

First utilized in oncology, radiomics has been successfully investigated to differentiate benign renal mass from malignancy and predict histopathology, survival, and outcome of various urologic cancers [13]. Radiomics aims to analyse and translate medical images into quantitative data and provide an image-based biomarker to aid clinical decisions and improve precision medicine [14]. Success in the oncologic field has drawn attention to the application of radiomics in benign urologic conditions, especially urolithiasis. An illustration of the workflow of radiomics in kidney stone disease is presented in Figure 1: (1) Image acquisition and pre-processing, (2) Validation and training dataset creation, (3) Extraction and feature segmentation, and (4) Model building, e.g., kidney stone analysis. Figure 2 illustrates the utility of radiomics when applied specifically to patients with kidney stone disease, with four potential key areas: (1) Diagnosis and prediction of pathological features in patients with kidney stone disease, (2) Risk stratification and prognosis of stone forming patients, (3) Categorisation and molecular profiling of high-risk stone formers; and (4) Implementation of personalized medicine in kidney stone formers.

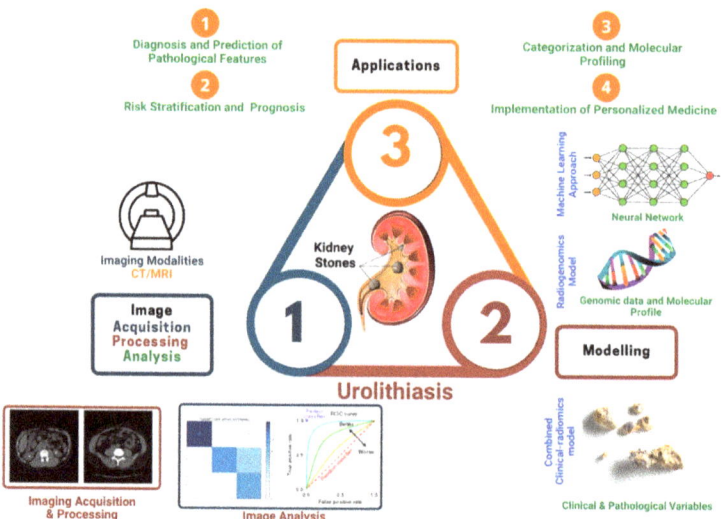

Figure 1. Potential contributions of radiomics and radiogenomics to the management of a patient with urolithiasis.

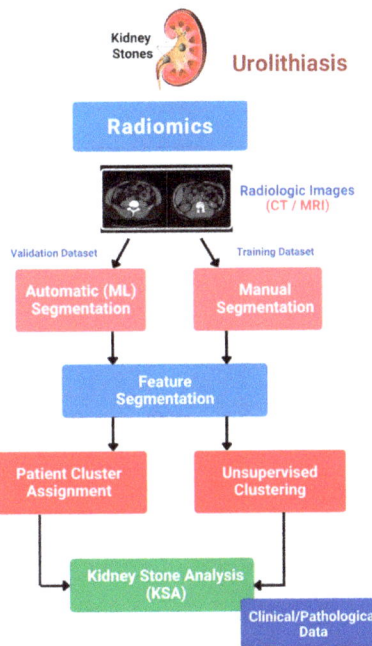

Figure 2. Radiomics approach in the treatment of patients with kidney stone disease.

The aim of the scoping review is to evaluate if radiomics-based applications can help endourologist overcome some confounders in stone management such as preoperative identification of stone composition, identifying phleboliths, and predicting stone free rate after medical expulsion therapy.

2. Materials and Methods

2.1. Literature Search

A literature review of the usage of radiomics in the setting of urolithiasis was performed using the Preferred Reporting Items for Systematic Reviews and Meta-Analyses (PRISMA) framework for scoping reviews and metanalysis guidelines. An electronic literature search was conducted on PubMed, EMBASE, and Scopus from inception to 21 March 2022 without language restrictions (Appendix A) [15]. The full search strategies are outlined in Appendix B. Abstracts and full texts retrieved were reviewed by two independent investigators; conflicts were resolved by a third author. The inclusion criteria were: (1) Use of radiomics in diagnostics, treatment prediction, or therapeutics; (2) Any type of urolithiasis, including nephrolithiasis, ureterolithiasis, and cystolithiasis. Case reports, abstracts, and reviews were excluded from the analysis. The data were extracted using a standardized data collection template with predefined data fields including study characteristics, objective of radiomics, study findings, and study conclusions.

2.2. Study Selection

The search strategy retrieved 1332 studies; after removal of 322 duplicates, the remaining 1010 studies were screened by title and abstract. Of the 108 studies shortlisted for full-text screening, 7 were eventually included in this review.

3. Results

The potential domains in which radiomics can contribute significantly are diagnostics, therapeutic, and interventional outcomes. A total of seven studies were included; one study by Perrot et al. [16] examined the use of radiomics in differentiating between phleboliths and calculi. Four studies reviewed identified stone type and composition, with two studies that looked at interventional outcomes [17,18]. Table 1 shows the included studies.

Table 1. Summary of included studies.

No.	Author (Year)	Type of Study	Objective	Number of Patients and Breakdown	Number of Radiomics Features	Utility	Conclusion
1	Perrot et al., (2022)	In-vivo	Identification of Urolithiasis	Training set: 369 patients (211 kidney stones, 201 phleboliths) Testing set: 43 patients (24 kidney stones, 23 phleboliths)	NR	Accuracy: 85.1% Sensitivity: 91.7% Specificity: 78.3% Positive predictive value: 81.5% Negative predictive value: 90.0% AUC: 0.902	Machine learning reinforced with machine learning enable accurate discernment between renal calculi and phleboliths on low-dose CT in patients with acute flank pain.
2	Cui et al., (2022)	In-vivo	Prediction of Stone Type	157 patients (98 infection kidney stones, 59 non-infection kidney stones)	54 radiomics features (16 morphological, 38 textural) → reduced to 27 key features (16 morphological, 11 textural) by the LASSO algorithm	Accuracy: 90.7% Sensitivity: 85.81% Specificity: 93.96% Positive predictive value: 91% Negative predictive value: 91% AUC: 0.97	Quantitative nomogram with radiomics method is useful for pre-operative prediction of infection versus non-infection kidney stones.
3	Zheng et al., (2022)	In-vivo	Prediction of Stone Type	Training set: 314 patients (41 infection stones, 273 non-infection stones) Internal validation set: 134 patients (22 infection stones, 112 non-infection stones) External validation set 1: 594 patients (111 infection stones, 483 non-infection stones) External validation set 2: 156 patients (18 infection stones, 138 non-infection stones)	1316 radiomics features → 24 key features with non-zero coefficients selected by the LASSO algorithm	Training set: AUC: 0.864 (95% CI 0.802–0.926) Internal validation set: 0.832 (95% CI 0.742–0.923) External validation set 1: 0.825 (95% CI 0.783–0.866) External validation set 2: 0.812 (95% CI 0.710–0.914)	Radiomics model developed can be a non-invasive method to detect urinary infection stones in vivo, benefitting subsequent management and patient prognosis.
4	Tang et al., (2022)	In-vivo	Prediction of Stone Composition	543 patients (373 calcium oxalate monohydrate stones, 170 non-COM stones)	1218 radiomics features extracted → 8 features with non-zero coefficients were selected for by the LASSO algorithm	Accuracy: 88.5% Sensitivity: 90.5% Specificity: 84.3% Training set AUC: 0.935 (95% CI 0.907–0.962) Testing set AUC: 0.933 (95% CI 0.893–0.973)	Artificial intelligence models incorporated with radiomics can predict COM and non-COM stones in vivo pre-operatively with robust accuracy, sensitivity, and specificity values.
5	Hameed et al., (2022)	In-vitro	Prediction of Stone Composition	NR	NR	Average accuracy: 87% Calcium oxalate monohydrate stone accuracy: 89% Calcium oxalate dihydrate stone accuracy: 85% Struvite stone accuracy: 86% Uric acid stone accuracy: 93% Calcium hydrogen phosphate stone accuracy: 89%	The artificial intelligence (deep learning-convolutional neural network DL-CNN) model reinforced with radiomics is successful in predicting various types of stone composition with high accuracy values.

Table 1. Cont.

No.	Author (Year)	Type of Study	Objective	Number of Patients and Breakdown	Number of Radiomics Features	Utility	Conclusion
6.	Xun et al., (2020)	In-vivo	PCNL: To develop and validate a novel clinical–radiomics nomogram model for pre-operatively predicting the stone-free rate of flexible ureteroscopy in patients with a single kidney stone	Training set: 99 patients Testing set (internal validation): 43 patients	Radiomics feature selection and signature building were conducted by using the least absolute shrinkage and selection operator (LASSO) method. With penalty parameter tuning conducted by 10-fold cross-validation, LASSO was performed to select robust and non-redundant features from the primary cohort. A radiomics signature was created by a linear combination of selected features weighted by their respective coefficients, and the relevant radiomics score was calculated for each patient.	AUC test group: 0.949 (95% CI, 0.910–0.989) AUC validation group: 0.947 (95% CI, 0.883–1)	Radiomics score, stone volume, hydronephrosis level, and operator experience were crucial for RIRS strategy
7.	Homayounieh et al., (2020)	In-vivo	RIRS: To assess if auto segmentation-assisted radiomics can predict disease burden, hydronephrosis, and treatment strategies in patients with renal calculi.	202 patients who underwent clinically indicated, non-contrast abdomen-pelvis CT for suspected or known renal calculi.	Deidentified CT images were processed with the radi-omics prototype (Radiomics, Frontier, Siemens Healthineers), which automatically segmented each kidney to obtain 1690 first-, shape-, and higher-order radiomics.	AUC: 0.91 (95% CI 0.85–0.92)	Automated segmentation and radiomics of entire kidneys can assess hydronephrosis presence, stone burden, and treatment strategies for renal calculi

NR: Not reported; AUC: Area under the curve; CT: Computed Tomography; PCNL: Percutaneous nephrolithotomy; RIRS: Retrograde intrarenal surgery.

4. Discussion

4.1. Diagnostics

4.1.1. Differentiating Ureteric Calculi and Phleboliths

First described in the 19th century, phleboliths generally present as layers of calcified fibrous tissue covered by a layer of endothelium which is continuous with the intimal layer of vein wall [19]. Differentiating characteristics include a central lucency, comet tail sign, and anatomical distribution [20]. Although advances in radiology have improved the landscape of differentiating phleboliths from ureteral calculi, they still present a diagnostic challenge particularly in the emergency setting, leading to unnecessary intervention and associated financial and resource burdens. Perrot et al. [16] sought to utilize the capabilities of radiomics to improve the use of low-dose unenhanced computed tomography (LDCT) in distinguishing renal calculi from pelvic phleboliths. The study involved independent training (369 patients, 211 kidney stones, and 201 phleboliths) and a testing cohort (43 patients, 24 kidney stones, and 23 phleboliths) for training and experimentation of the machine-learning classifier, respectively. Both patient groups presented with acute renal colic and subsequently underwent LDCT for radiological assessment. A total of 147,029 radiomics features (first-order, shape, gray level co-occurrence matrix (GLCM), gray level size zone matrix (GLSZM), gray level run length matrix (GLRLM), neighboring gray-tone difference matrix (NGTDM), and gray level dependence matrix (GLDM)) extracted from LDCT images were used for prediction by the model, demonstrating an overall accuracy of 85.1%, 91.7% sensitivity, and 78.3% specificity with a ROC-AUC value of 0.902. This radiomics-reinforced machine-learning algorithm proves itself to be a highly objective method for discerning renal calculi and might be helpful in limiting unnecessary interventions.

4.1.2. Pre-Operative Identification of Stone Type

Radiomics features have also been employed to guide the detection of calculi material, largely within the pre-operative context to guide downstream management. Cui et al. [21] developed a radiomics signature created with ensemble learning based on bagged trees and applied it to non-contrast CT images of 157 patients diagnosed with either infection stone (98 patients) or non-infection stone (59 patients). With the least absolute shrinkage and selection operator (LASSO) algorithm, 27 radiomics features with the highest predictabilities were selected. The model reported 90.7% accuracy, 85.8% sensitivity, and 94.0% specificity with a ROC value of 0.97 in determining the presence of infection kidney stones. In the same vein, Zheng et al. [22] established a radiomics-signature incorporated radiomics model after extraction of data from CT images of 1198 urolithiasis patients, with 24 best radiomics features finalized by LASSO from 1316 radiomics features. AUC values of 0.898 (95% CI 0.840–0.956), 0.832 (95% CI 0.742–0.923), 0.825 (95% CI 0.783–0.866), and 0.812 (95% CI 0.710–0.914) were attained with the model on training and validation cohorts. The model also performed significantly better ($p < 0.001$) than urine pH, urine white blood cell count, urine nitrite, and presence of urease-producing bacteria in determining the existence of infection renal stones.

Tang et al. [23] specifically looked at the prediction of the occurrence of calcium oxalate monohydrate (COM) stones, the most prevalent stone type in routine practice. A total of 1218 radiomics features were extracted from 337 COM and 107 non-COM calculi seen on pre-operative non-contrast CT images, and 8 with non-zero coefficients were selected for the model by LASSO. Incorporation into the AI model revealed an accuracy, sensitivity, and specificity of 88.5%, 90.5%, and 84.3%, respectively, with an AUC value of 0.935 (95% CI 0.907–0.962) in the training cohort and 0.933 (95% CI 0.893–0.973) in the testing set for pre-operative prediction of COM vs. non-COM stones. Hameed et al. [24] applied deep learning convolutional neural network (DLCNN) guided by radiomics features demonstrating 87% accuracy of prediction of calculi type. Specificity of each type of calculi was 89% for COM stones, 85% for calcium oxalate dihydrate stones, 86% for struvite stones, 93% for uric acid stones, and 89% for calcium hydrogen phosphate stones. However, despite improvements with added anatomical location and the ability to aid in differentiating between pelvic phleboliths and ureteric calculi, there are still sizable inaccuracies if artificial intelligence is used alone. Like AI, radiomics too can efficiently process vast quantities of data. With the shift towards electronic patient records, increasingly more big data sets are created and this will allow AI and radiomics to analyse and detect novel diagnostic and treatment patterns in the future [25].

Summary: With increasing application and accuracy of radiomics in differentiating phleboliths from true calculi and stone type, this can potentially influence the choice of treatment modality and limit unnecessary surgical intervention with its associated financial burden and morbidity.

4.2. Evaluating Treatment Outcomes

Radiomics has been also applied in the field of urolithiasis to predict the complications and outcomes of endourological procedures. We review their role in the various treatment modalities in predicting treatment efficacy.

4.2.1. Prediction of Spontaneous Stone Passage

Radiomics has also been applied to predict spontaneous stone passage rate in symptomatic patients. Mohammadinejad et al. compared the ability of a semi-automated radiomics analysis software in predicting the likelihood of spontaneous stone passage with manual measurements. Stone characteristics including length, width, height, maximal diameter, volume, the mean and standard deviation of the Hounsfield units, and morphologic features were extracted from CT images using automated radiomics analysis software [26]. Univariate analysis and multivariate analysis showed AUC of 0.82 and 0.83, respectively, for maximum stone diameter measured manually. The AUC for a model including automatic measurement of maximum height and diameter of the stone was

0.82. Hence, the authors concluded that semi-automated radiomics analysis shows similar accuracy compared with manual measurements in predicting spontaneous stone passage.

4.2.2. Therapeutic Utility in ESWL

Despite numerous AI-based platforms exploring the utility of decision algorithms in ESWL, there were no articles that focused specifically on radiomics devised applications for ESWL, proving it to be uncharted therapy. It will be interesting to continue to monitor if refined technologies such as burst wave lithotripsy will fuel renewed interest in the application of radiomics in this modality of treatment [27].

4.2.3. Predicting Stone Burden Affecting RIRS/PCNL Stone-Free Rates Outcomes

The application of radiomics in endourology is relatively novel, and only two reports have been so far published, one in PCNL [17] and the second one in RIRS [18]. Homayounieh et al. analysed 202 kidney stone adult patients who underwent CT scan for evaluation of renal colic or stones in three different CT machines [2]. The purpose of this study was to assess if an automatically segmented whole renal radiomics was able to estimate the stone burden and predict hydronephrosis and treatment strategies from CT images. All stone images were evaluated by a single experienced radiologist who assessed manually the stone location and burden (stone density, stone size, and stone contours) and the presence or not of hydronephrosis for each patient. A physician expert in image processing processed all CT examinations from a standalone radiomics prototype that automatically recognized and segmented the entire kidney volume, including all stones included within the segmentation contours. After confirmation of the contours, the radiomics prototype estimated 1690 first-, shape, and higher-order radiomics for each kidney. Among the 202 patients, the radiomics prototype was able to discriminate between patients with and without renal stones (AUC 0.84, 95% CI 0.78–0.89, $p < 0.003$). Radiomics was also able to accurately detect hydronephrosis (AUC 0.89, 95% CI 0.8–0.89, $p < 0.003$). In addition, radiomics was able to predict patients managed with PCNL. Stone burden in these patients was significantly larger than those managed conservatively (641 $\pm$ 1090 vs. 53 $\pm$ 8 mm^3, $p < 0.0001$). Interestingly, there was no difference in radiomics vendors performance between the three CT machines across all study outcomes. The automatic segmentation and inclusion of the entire kidney volume enabled the authors to apply radiomics not only to the stone but to the whole renal volume to obtain a consistent and generalizable prediction of stone burden and the need for PCNL treatment.

Factors such as location [28], size and volume of stone burden [29,30], and Hounsfield units (HU) [31] are key determinants and predictors of stone-free rates in both normal and anomalous kidneys alike [32,33]. Stone size limits the use of HU for the prediction of stone composition, especially calcium oxalate stones, and is a known limitation for predicting successful outcomes in ESWL and PCNL [34,35] Xun et al. retrospectively assessed 264 patients with a solitary kidney stone who underwent RIRS [18]. Among these, 142 patients had a lower calix stone. Preoperative assessment was made with an unenhanced 64-slice CT scan. Stones were manually segmented on each transverse slice CT image. Radiomics feature extraction was accomplished operating an in-house texture analysis software, including a total of 604 radiomics features (first-order statistics, shape- and size-based features, textural features, and wavelet features) generated from each original CT image. A radiomics signature was generated by a linear combination of selected features weighted by their respective coefficients, and a radiomics score (Rad-score) was estimated for each patient. Finally, the authors developed a visual nomogram incorporating clinical and radiomics parameters to predict SFR, defined as residual fragments less than 2 mm. Interestingly, radiomics score significantly differed between SFR and non-SFR patients both in the test and validation group with higher scores observed in patients with higher SFR. The prediction nomogram was very accurate (AUC 0.94, 95% CI, 0.910–0.989) and its predictive efficacy was confirmed by the validation group (AUC 0.947, 95% CI 0.883–1). The inclusion of radiomics in this model demonstrated to be an effective preoperative prediction method for clinical decision-making in patients undergoing RIRS. The main advantage of using radiomics in this context relies mostly on the speed of the procedure in a more quantitative and reproducible manner as compared with the manual assessment which can be time-consuming and prone to intra and interobserver variations, particularly for complex renal stones requiring a PCNL treatment (i.e., staghorn and multiple stones) [36].

Summary: This adds a significant research potential wherein using the radiomics signatures comparisons can be made between the efficacy of single emission CT scans (SECT) vis a vis dual emission CT scans to accurately determine stone composition [37]. This information can enable endourologists to better choose the right intervention for their patient and potentially overcome limitations and act as adjuncts of various scoring systems used as surrogate tools for predicting success in endourology interventions [38].

4.3. Current Limitations and Future Directions

One limitation of deep learning-based radiomics is the dependent correlation between the features and the input data, as the features are generated from that very dataset. Therefore, in contrast to feature-based radiomics, large datasets are necessary to accurately identify the relevant and robust feature subsets. This limitation can be partially overcome by utilizing a machine learning technique called transfer learning, by using a pre-trained neural network on a different but similarly related task, e.g., Neural data that was trained to predict renal stones can also be used and trained on how to measure and classify residual fragments after a procedure [39]. Another limitation is the reproducibility and transferability of radiomics features as it is heavily dependent on size, quality, sequence, modality, resolution, and motion artifacts of image transfer; Traverso et al. performed a recent review and identified radiomics features that were reproducible and repeatable [40]. Moving forward, the Image Biomarker Standardization Initiative (IBSI) has been established to provide standardized image biomarker nomenclature and definition, as well as to aid in formulating reporting guidelines to regulate effective communication and verification within study groups in the field of radiomics [41]. These principles when applied to the field of radiomics for urolithiasis could help standardize and refine accessibility, facilitating a widespread acceptance of the same. Xun et al. developed and validated a clinical-radiomics nomogram model for pre-operatively predicting the stone free rate of flexible ureteroscopy. They demonstrated that when applied, radiomics scores from their nomogram had satisfactory predictive accuracy in clinical application [18]. Radiomics may be used in the future to generate or validate nomograms that aid in accessing or predicting stone-free rates based on the modality of intervention.

4.4. Take Home Messages

In summary, potential applications of radiomics in urolithiasis are:
1. Predicting success of spontaneous stone passage with medical expulsion therapy.
2. Differentiating between calculi and phleboliths.
3. Pre-operative accurate identification of stone type.
4. Predicting stone burden affecting RIRS/PCNL stone-free rate outcomes.

5. Conclusions

Our review shows that radiomics in urolithiasis is still in infancy. Its best potential lies in identifying infectious stones preoperatively; whether this application can extend to all stone types remains undetermined. Future applications in ESWL and predicting stone free rates for different compositions are the next frontiers for research and development. It is hoped that with further correlation of radiomics with conventional established sources of diagnostic subsets such as clinical, molecular, and imaging can optimize disease management in urolithiasis and improve patient prognosis.

Author Contributions: Conceptualization, E.J.L., D.C., C.T.H., B.S. and V.G.; Data curation, N.N. and K.S.; Formal analysis, E.J.L. and K.S.; Funding acquisition, H.Y.T.; Investigation, W.Z.S. and J.Y.-C.T.; Methodology, E.J.L. and K.Y.F.; Project administration, H.Y.T., N.G., J.D.L.R., B.S. and V.G.; Resources, C.T.H., K.G. and V.G.; Software, K.Y.F. and K.G.; Supervision, J.Y.-C.T., N.N. and K.S.; Visualization, J.Q.L.; Writing—original draft, E.J.L., D.C., W.Z.S. and J.Q.L.; Writing—review & editing, H.Y.T., N.G., J.D.L.R., B.S. and V.G. All authors have read and agreed to the published version of the manuscript.

Funding: This research received no external funding.

Institutional Review Board Statement: Not applicable.

Informed Consent Statement: Not applicable.

Data Availability Statement: Not applicable.

Conflicts of Interest: The authors declare no conflict of interest.

Appendix A

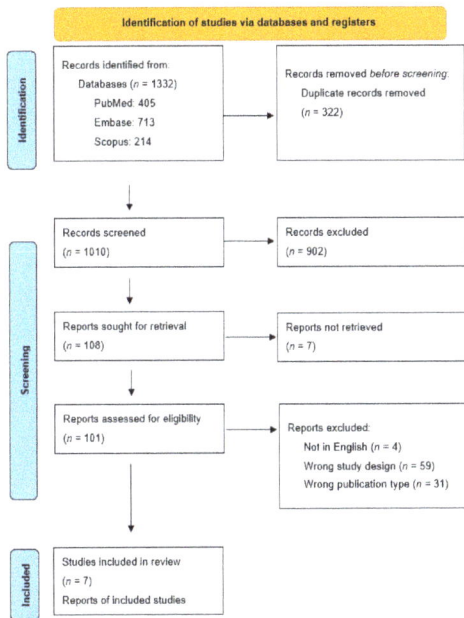

Figure A1. PRISMA 2020 Flow Diagram.

Appendix B

Table A1. Full search phrases used for the respective databases.

PubMed	405 Articles
((stone * AND (renal OR kidney OR ureter OR ureteric OR bladder)) OR ('Urolithiasis' [MeSH]) OR ('Calculi' [MeSH]) OR ('Kidney Calculi' [MeSH]) OR nephrolithiasis OR ureterolithiasis OR cystolithiasis) AND ("artificial intelligence" [MeSH] OR "AI" OR "radiomic *" OR "machine learning" OR "deep learning")	
EMBASE	**713 articles**
((stone OR stones) AND (renal OR kidney OR ureter OR ureteric OR bladder) OR 'urolithiasis'/exp OR 'calculi'/exp OR 'nephrolithiasis'/exp OR 'ureterolithiasis'/exp OR cystolithiasis) AND ('artificial intelligence'/exp OR 'ai' OR 'radiomic' OR 'radiomics'/exp OR 'machine learning'/exp OR 'deep learning')	
Scopus	**214 articles**
TITLE-ABS-KEY (((stone OR stones OR calculi OR calculus AND (renal OR kidney OR ureter OR ureteric OR bladder)) OR urolithiasis OR nephrolithiasis OR ureterolithiasis OR cystolithiasis) AND ("artificial intelligence" OR "AI" OR "radiomic" OR "radiomics" OR "machine learning" OR "deep learning"))	

Date searched: 21 March 2022. Pre-deduplication 1332. Post-deduplication 1010.

References

1. Rajpurkar, P.; Chen, E.; Banerjee, O.; Topol, E.J. AI in health and medicine. *Nat. Med.* **2022**, *28*, 31–38. [CrossRef]
2. Vailati-Riboni, M.; Palombo, V.; Loor, J.J. *What are Omics Sciences? Periparturient Diseases of Dairy Cows*; Springer: Berlin/Heidelberg, Germany, 2017; pp. 1–7. [CrossRef]
3. Lambin, P.; Rios-Velazquez, E.; Leijenaar, R.; Carvalho, S.; van Stiphout, R.G.P.M.; Granton, P.; Zegers, C.M.L.; Gillies, R.; Boellard, R.; Dekker, A.; et al. Radiomics: Extracting more information from medical images using advanced feature analysis. *Eur. J. Cancer* **2012**, *48*, 441–446. [CrossRef]
4. Van Timmeren, J.E.; Cester, D.; Tanadini-Lang, S.; Alkadhi, H.; Baessler, B. Radiomics in medical imaging—"How-to" guide and critical reflection. *Insights Imaging* **2020**, *11*, 91. [CrossRef] [PubMed]
5. Mills, S.; Irakliotis, L.; Carlson, T.; Lucas, S.; Perlowitz, B. Demystifying Big Data: A Practical Guide to Transforming the Business of Government. Available online: https://bigdatawg.nist.gov/_uploadfiles/M0068_v1_3903747095.pdf (accessed on 13 August 2022).
6. Castellano, G.; Bonilha, L.; Li, L.M.; Cendes, F. Texture analysis of medical images. *Clin. Radiol.* **2004**, *59*, 1061–1069. [CrossRef]
7. Tourassi, G.D. Journey toward computer-aided diagnosis: Role of image texture analysis. *Radiology* **1999**, *213*, 317–320. [CrossRef] [PubMed]
8. Wagner, M.W.; Namdar, K.; Biswas, A.; Monah, S.; Khalvati, F.; Ertl-Wagner, B.B. Radiomics, machine learning, and artificial intelligence—What the neuroradiologist needs to know. *Neuroradiology* **2021**, *63*, 1957–1967. [CrossRef] [PubMed]
9. Gillies, R.J.; Kinahan, P.E.; Hricak, H. Radiomics: Images Are More than Pictures, They Are Data. *Radiology* **2016**, *278*, 563–577. [CrossRef]
10. Rizzo, S.; Botta, F.; Raimondi, S.; Origgi, D.; Fanciullo, C.; Morganti, A.G.; Bellomi, M. Radiomics: The facts and the challenges of image analysis. *Eur. Radiol. Exp.* **2018**, *2*, 36. [CrossRef]
11. Cho, H.; Lee, H.Y.; Kim, E.; Lee, G.; Kim, J.; Kwon, J.; Park, H. Radiomics-guided deep neural networks stratify lung adenocarcinoma prognosis from CT scans. *Commun. Biol.* **2021**, *4*, 1–12. [CrossRef]
12. Zhang, X.; Zhang, Y.; Zhang, G.; Qiu, X.; Tan, W.; Yin, X.; Liao, L. Deep Learning with Radiomics for Disease Diagnosis and Treatment: Challenges and Potential. *Front. Oncol.* **2022**, *12*, 773840. [CrossRef]
13. Scrivener, M.; de Jong, E.E.C.; van Timmeren, J.; Pieters, T.; Ghaye, B.; Geets, X. Radiomics applied to lung cancer: A review. *Transl. Cancer Res.* **2016**, *5*, 398–409. [CrossRef]
14. Avanzo, M.; Stancanello, J.; El Naqa, I. Beyond imaging: The promise of radiomics. *Phys. Med.* **2017**, *38*, 122–139. [CrossRef] [PubMed]
15. Page, M.J.; McKenzie, J.E.; Bossuyt, P.M.; Boutron, I.; Hoffmann, T.C.; Mulrow, C.D.; Shamseer, L.; Tetzlaff, J.M.; Akl, E.A.; Brennan, S.E.; et al. The PRISMA 2020 statement: An updated guideline for reporting systematic reviews. *PLOS Med.* **2021**, *18*, e1003583. [CrossRef] [PubMed]
16. De Perrot, T.; Hofmeister, J.; Burgermeister, S.; Martin, S.P.; Feutry, G.; Klein, J.; Montet, X. Differentiating kidney stones from phleboliths in unenhanced low-dose computed tomography using radiomics and machine learning. *Eur. Radiol.* **2019**, *29*, 4776–4782. [CrossRef]
17. Homayounieh, F.; Doda Khera, R.; Bizzo, B.C.; Ebrahimian, S.; Primak, A.; Schmidt, B.; Saini, S.; Kalra, M.K. Prediction of burden and management of renal calculi from whole kidney radiomics: A multicenter study. *Abdom. Radiol.* **2021**, *46*, 2097–2106. [CrossRef] [PubMed]

18. Xun, Y.; Chen, M.; Liang, P.; Tripathi, P.; Deng, H.; Zhou, Z.; Xie, Q.; Li, C.; Wang, S.; Li, Z.; et al. A Novel Clinical-Radiomics Model Pre-operatively Predicted the Stone-Free Rate of Flexible Ureteroscopy Strategy in Kidney Stone Patients. *Front. Med.* **2020**, *7*, 576925. [CrossRef]
19. Luk, A.C.O.; Cleaveland, P.; Olson, L.; Neilson, D.; Srirangam, S.J. Pelvic Phlebolith: A Trivial Pursuit for the Urologist? *J. Endourol.* **2017**, *31*, 342–347. [CrossRef]
20. Carius, B.M.; Long, B. Is This Your Stone? Distinguishing Phleboliths and Nephroliths on Imaging in the Emergency Department Setting. *J. Emerg. Med.* **2022**, *62*, 316–323. [CrossRef]
21. Cui, X.; Che, F.; Wang, N.; Liu, X.; Zhu, Y.; Zhao, Y.; Bi, J.; Li, Z.; Zhang, G. Preoperative Prediction of Infection Stones Using Radiomics Features from Computed Tomography. *IEEE Access* **2019**, *7*, 122675–122683. [CrossRef]
22. Zheng, J.; Yu, H.; Batur, J.; Shi, Z.; Tuerxun, A.; Abulajiang, A.; Lu, S.; Kong, J.; Huang, L.; Wu, S.; et al. A multicenter study to develop a non-invasive radiomic model to identify urinary infection stone in vivo using machine-learning. *Kidney Int.* **2021**, *100*, 870–880. [CrossRef]
23. Tang, L.; Li, W.; Zeng, X.; Wang, R.; Yang, X.; Luo, G.; Chen, Q.; Wang, L.; Song, B. Value of artificial intelligence model based on unenhanced computed tomography of urinary tract for preoperative prediction of calcium oxalate monohydrate stones in vivo. *Ann. Transl. Med.* **2021**, *9*, 1129. [CrossRef] [PubMed]
24. Hameed, B.M.Z.; Somani, B.; Naik, N.; Talasila, A.; Shah, M.; Reddy, S.; Sachdev, G.; Hussein Beary, R.; Hegde, P. Application of deep learning convolutional neural network in prediction of stone location, skin to stone distance and composition in renal lithiasis: A single center pilot study. *Eur. Urol.* **2021**, *79*, S336. [CrossRef]
25. Yang, B.; Veneziano, D.; Somani, B.K. Artificial intelligence in the diagnosis, treatment and prevention of urinary stones. *Curr. Opin. Urol.* **2020**, *30*, 782–787. [CrossRef] [PubMed]
26. Mohammadinejad, P.; Ferrero, A.; Bartlett, D.J.; Khandelwal, A.; Marcus, R.; Lieske, J.C.; Moen, T.R.; Mara, K.C.; Enders, F.T.; McCollough, C.H.; et al. Automated radiomic analysis of CT images to predict likelihood of spontaneous passage of symptomatic renal stones. *Emerg. Radiol.* **2021**, *28*, 781–788. [CrossRef] [PubMed]
27. Maxwell, A.D.; Wang, Y.-N.; Kreider, W.; Cunitz, B.W.; Starr, F.; Lee, D.; Nazari, Y.; Williams, J.C., Jr.; Bailey, M.R.; Sorensen, M.D. Evaluation of Renal Stone Comminution and Injury by Burst Wave Lithotripsy in a Pig Model. *J. Endourol.* **2019**, *33*, 787–792. [CrossRef]
28. Bhanot, R.; Jones, P.; Somani, B. Minimally Invasive Surgery for the Treatment of Ureteric Stones—State-of-the-Art Review. *Res. Rep. Urol.* **2021**, *13*, 227–236. [CrossRef]
29. Karim, S.S.; Hanna, L.; Geraghty, R.; Somani, B.K. Role of pelvicalyceal anatomy in the outcomes of retrograde intrarenal surgery (RIRS) for lower pole stones: Outcomes with a systematic review of literature. *Urolithiasis* **2020**, *48*, 263–270. [CrossRef]
30. Reddy, T.G.; Assimos, D.G. Optimizing Stone-free Rates with Ureteroscopy. *Rev. Urol.* **2015**, *17*, 160–164.
31. Ermis, O.; Somani, B.; Reeves, T.; Guven, S.; Pes, P.L.; Chawla, A.; Hegde, P.; de la Rosette, J. Definition, treatment and outcome of residual fragments in staghorn stones. *Asian J. Urol.* **2020**, *7*, 116–121. [CrossRef]
32. Lim, E.J.; Teoh, J.Y.; Fong, K.Y.; Emiliani, E.; Gadzhiev, N.; Gorelov, D.; Tanidir, Y.; Sepulveda, F.; Al-Terki, A.; Khadgi, S.; et al. Propensity score-matched analysis comparing retrograde intrarenal surgery with percutaneous nephrolithotomy in anomalous kidneys. *Minerva Urol. Nephrol.* **2022**. [CrossRef]
33. García Rojo, E.; Teoh, J.Y.-C.; Castellani, D.; Brime Menéndez, R.; Tanidir, Y.; Benedetto Galosi, A.; Bhatia, T.P.; Soebhali, B.; Sridharan, V.; Corrales, M.; et al. Real-world Global Outcomes of Retrograde Intrarenal Surgery in Anomalous Kidneys: A High Volume International Multicenter Study. *Urology* **2022**, *159*, 41–47. [CrossRef] [PubMed]
34. Gok, A.; Polat, H.; Cift, A.; Yucel, M.O.; Gok, B.; Sirik, M.; Benlioglu, C.; Kalyenci, B. The hounsfield unit value calculated with the aid of non-contrast computed tomography and its effect on the outcome of percutaneous nephrolithotomy. *Urolithiasis* **2015**, *43*, 277–281. [CrossRef] [PubMed]
35. Stewart, G.; Johnson, L.; Ganesh, H.; Davenport, D.; Smelser, W.; Crispen, P.; Venkatesh, R. Stone Size Limits the Use of Hounsfield Units for Prediction of Calcium Oxalate Stone Composition. *Urology* **2015**, *85*, 292–295. [CrossRef] [PubMed]
36. Selby, M.G.; Vrtiska, T.J.; Krambeck, A.E.; McCollough, C.H.; Elsherbiny, H.E.; Bergstralh, E.J.; Lieske, J.C.; Rule, A.D. Quantification of asymptomatic kidney stone burden by computed tomography for predicting future symptomatic stone events. *Urology* **2015**, *85*, 45–50. [CrossRef]
37. Wisenbaugh, E.S.; Paden, R.G.; Silva, A.C.; Humphreys, M.R. Dual-energy vs conventional computed tomography in determining stone composition. *Urology* **2014**, *83*, 1243–1247. [CrossRef]
38. Jones, P.; Pietropaolo, A.; Chew, B.H.; Somani, B.K. Atlas of Scoring Systems, Grading Tools, and Nomograms in Endourology: A Comprehensive Overview from the TOWER Endourological Society Research Group. *J. Endourol.* **2021**, *35*, 1863–1882. [CrossRef]
39. Lohmann, P.; Bousabarah, K.; Hoevels, M.; Treuer, H. Radiomics in radiation oncology—Basics, methods, and limitations. *Strahlenther Onkol.* **2020**, *196*, 848–855. [CrossRef]
40. Traverso, A.; Wee, L.; Dekker, A.; Gillies, R. Repeatability and Reproducibility of Radiomic Features: A Systematic Review. *Int. J. Radiat. Oncol. Biol. Phys.* **2018**, *102*, 1143–1158. [CrossRef]
41. Zwanenburg, A.; Vallières, M.; Abdalah, M.A.; Aerts, H.J.W.L.; Andrearczyk, V.; Apte, A.; Ashrafinia, S.; Bakas, S.; Beukinga, R.J.; Boellaard, R.; et al. The Image Biomarker Standardization Initiative: Standardized Quantitative Radiomics for High-Throughput Image-based Phenotyping. *Radiology* **2020**, *295*, 328–338. [CrossRef]

MDPI
St. Alban-Anlage 66
4052 Basel
Switzerland
Tel. +41 61 683 77 34
Fax +41 61 302 89 18
www.mdpi.com

Journal of Clinical Medicine Editorial Office
E-mail: jcm@mdpi.com
www.mdpi.com/journal/jcm

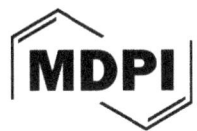

www.ingramcontent.com/pod-product-compliance
Lightning Source LLC
LaVergne TN
LVHW070554100526
838202LV00012B/462